BEFORE THE END OF THE DAY

...And before the end of the day
we were scattered like stars or like rain
and all this must come to an end
and never again to be met with...

— Li Po   (7th Century A.D.)

Before the End of the Day

STORIES FROM A DOCTOR'S JOURNAL

Michael Malus

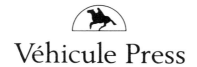

Véhicule Press

Published with the assistance of The Canada Council.

The author wishes to thank publisher Simon Dardick and editor Vicki Marcok for their warm reception of my manuscript and their firm and caring hand in its birth as a book.

Cover art: J.W. Stewart
Design and imaging: Simon Garamond
Printing: Imprimerie d'Édition Marquis Ltée

Dépôt légal, Bibliothèque nationale du Québec and the National Library of Canada, fourth quarter 1994.

CANADIAN CATALOGUING IN PUBLICATION DATA
Malus, Michael
   Before the end of the day : stories from
a doctor's journal.
ISBN: 1-55065-055-6
   1. Malus, Michael   2. Physicians—Northwest Territories—Great Slave Lake—Biography. 3.Physicians—Hudson Bay—Biography. 4. Physicians—Quebec (Province)—Biography.
5. Physicians—New Mexico—Mescalero.
6. Mescalero Indian Reservations, N.M.   I. Title.

R464.M35A3 1994   610'.92   C94-900854-0

Published by Véhicule Press, P.O.B. 125, Place du Parc Station, Montréal, Québec, Canada H2W 2M9.

Distributed in Canada by General Publishing, and in the United States by Inland Book Company.

Printed in Canada on acid-free paper.

Especially for Elaine,
Eli and Shem

Contents

AUTHOR'S NOTE

These stories are drawn from actual experiences I have had working as a doctor. The trust accorded to a physician by his patients is the starting point in the adventure that every clinical encounter unfolds. It allows the doctor the privilege of witnessing the dignity, courage, warmth and humour that patients so often reveal when that trust is assured. It is in this spirit that the names of people and places have been changed to protect identity, privacy and medical confidence.

Sunrise

Sunrise

Moe's River
4:45 a.m.

MY ALARM CLOCK has been ringing at four forty-five in the morning for years. I can't really say I'm used to it. Each morning I'm still horrified to hear it. I know if I say to myself *I'll just lie here another minute*, I'll fall back to sleep and wake up in about two hours. So I struggle up immediately and wash my face in cold water to really wake up.

Usually I've only had about five hours sleep. Even after washing my face and settling down in front of the typewriter the urge to jump back into bed is strong. My need for the calm and solitude of early morning keeps me from doing it. Being a country doctor with my office in my home, I won't know silence from eight in the morning until after ten or eleven at night. The telephone will ring at least ten times an hour, and the doorbell four or five. But now it's quiet. Someone may come with a pain in the belly or an earache. One of my pregnant patients may go into labour. But chances are I will have the next two hours for writing this journal.

I set the alarm at a quarter to five because the first fifteen minutes goes to starting a fire in the woodstove. That gives me two hours until seven, when I have to wake the family and help get the kids ready for the school bus which comes at eight. By that time there are always two or three patients sitting in the waiting room. With an hour break for lunch, which most often ends up as fifteen minutes, I usually have seen about thirty or forty patients by six at night. I don't schedule patients after supper, but being a doctor in an isolated area, where the nearest hospital is thirty miles away, between supper and ten or eleven at night there will be at least four or five more people calling with problems which are emergencies. Often they come without calling.

Between seeing these patients at night, I return non-urgent phone calls from earlier in the day, phone patients to see how they're doing, phone the relatives of patients in the hospital, read letters from consultants about patients I've referred and write to them about others, re-read relevant information in my medical books about diseases I'm treating, and read an article or two from a medical journal. Invariably, by the time I've cleared off my desk and straightened up the office, it's midnight.

All this is in no way a complaint. I love being a doctor. I take pride in it and feel privileged to be doing it. I feel a sense of adventure each time I see a patient. This description of my day is not a lament. I'm just explaining why the only time I have to write in this journal is from five to seven in the morning.

Our home is a farm situated about five miles from a town called Moe's River, and three miles from a village called St-Mathias-de-Bonneterre. We keep chickens and pigs and a large vegetable garden. When I say we, I really mean my wife Lenore. She maintains the farm with little help from me because of the demands of my medical practice. We also have a few head of beef cattle. These are cared for by our neighbour, Réjean, who is a dairy farmer. We give him space in our barn to keep some of his cattle in exchange for work he does for us.

Réjean is a forty-five year old bachelor who seems to go about his life making less mistakes than most people; or at least when he makes one, he doesn't repeat it. He is an extraordinarily dependable person. I rely on him totally for the upkeep of the farm. On the other hand he relies on me for the medical care of his aging parents. For years his mother had suffered from attacks of dizziness and weakness. They had been called psychological, and she had been treated unsuccessfully with anti-depressant medication. Simply because I live close by, I was able to examine her during one of the attacks of dizziness, and found that she had an intermittent disturbance in her heart rate that was the cause. Since that day she's been on medicine which prevents these attacks. I've helped his father through two episodes of severe pneumonia. The father also has cancer of the stomach. Again, because I was close by, and he came to me at an early stage, he has had no recurrence of the tumour since his operation three years ago. If he reaches five years without recurrence, it means he's home free.

A mutual respect for each other's ability forms the basis for a good relation between Réjean and me. It's been years now that we've been meeting on the run. Réjean also gets up at five to get his day's work done. When we stop and talk, an endless mental list of as yet undone farming chores looms over him, and the bottomlesss round of medical tasks I've just described beckons me. Despite this sense of distraction inherent in almost all our meetings, a deep friendship has been forged. We're always glad to see each other. His competence in farming aside, Réjean is an astute observer of people. I savour his observations. For example, there was his summary remark about René Cyr, a neighbour he had known for twenty years.

René was a nervous, chain-smoking man in his early fifties who owned the farm between Réjean and me. His farming was minimal; he supported himself by woodcutting. He worked hard, and was a good husband and father to his nine children. He always looked worried and harried — the one exception was once when I'd seen him on a Sunday at his house. I was over there seeing one of the kids who was sick. He was playing cards with some of the older boys at the kitchen table after dinner and he was relaxed and smiling. I had never seen that side of him, and was glad to see he could unwind.

One morning when he was gone to get the mail, his wife noticed that he was taking a long time. The mailbox was at the roadside about a hundred yards from the house. She looked out the window and saw him lying in the snow beside the box. She ran out to find him writhing from pain in his chest. He was pale and sweating, and could barely speak. She half dragged and half carried René to the house. At that time I hadn't yet started my office on the farm, and was working in a clinic thirty miles away. She called the doctor in Moe's River and asked him to come to the house. The doctor said it sounded like indigestion and told her to bring him to the office. One of the sons had taken the pick-up truck a half a mile down the road to where he and the father were currently logging. The mother sent the seven year old to get him. In parking the truck at the logging site, the son had put it too far into deep snow. It took him twenty minutes of digging and rocking the truck back and forth to get it out.

The doctor examined René and said he'd probably had a heart attack. He gave him an injection for pain, and called for an ambulance from the regional medical centre thirty miles away. An hour later the ambulance still hadn't come. The doctor suggested the family take him themselves. There was no room for him to lie down in the pick-up truck, so they waited another fifteen minutes for René's brother, who had a station wagon in which René could lie down.

On the way to the hospital a long freight train delayed them twelve minutes at a railway crossing. He died four minutes away from the hospital. When we were discussing René's death, Réjean said:

"He died as he lived—in a hurry."

Similarly, there was his succinct, epitaphic observation on the life and death of Madame Mathilde Arcand.

She lived down the road from us with her husband in a two-room shack in the tiny village of St-Mathias-de-Bonneterre. The village consists of several houses clustered along the road beside a church and a general store. Its population is about two hundred.

Our farm is situated between St-Mathias and Moe's River, about two miles closer to St-Mathias. Because Moe's River is larger and better known than St-Mathias, I'm generally referred to as the doctor from Moe's River. But, of course, the people from St-Mathias steadfastedly refer to me as the doctor from St-Mathias. Country towns are dying out in Quebec, and so are country doctors. Because of lack of work, many of the young people are moving to the cities. St-Mathias no longer has sufficient children to support a village school. The school is now an empty rotting building, and the children are bussed to school in a larger town thirty miles away. For the people of St-Mathias, to be able to say they had a doctor was like saying the village was alive and well. My presence itself was therapeutic. My mere appearance in Louis-Phillipe Dumont's general store was a remedial act. Any word I spoke was like an injection of the town's lost vitality. Anyway, back to Madame Mathilde Arcand and Réjean's summary remark about her death. She was about seventy-five years old when she died. Her husband's name is Cléophas. He's about eighty-five. He is one of the few people in St-Mathias who speaks English. Though I speak French as well as he speaks English, he is immensely proud of his English and insists on using it with me. He would call me about every three or four months, when his arthritis was a little worse than usual. He also had a duodenal ulcer which never really healed, because he could never give up the large amount of whisky he drank daily. When Cléophas smiles, he looks like a skeleton being reborn as a stubble-faced infant content after a feeding. His rasping voice on the telephone has the same uplifting quality as his smile. Since he's eighty-five, and has arthritis, and finds my stairs difficult, I always see him at his house. The visit itself is all I really have to offer in the way of treatment. There's not very much to do for the combination of arthritis and ulcer in an eighty-five year old. To begin with, all the medicines for controlling arthritis can cause ulcers, or at least make them worse. All I could give him for the arthritis was medicine for pain. As far as his ulcer was concerned, he drank bottles of whisky and chalky white antacids alternately, and took another medicine that diminished acid secretion in the stomach. The medicines would never really help him unless he stopped drinking, which we both knew he would never do.

On each visit his wife Mathilde would ask me to take her blood pressure. It was always normal. She had no medical complaints. Her only single complaint was a social one, never voiced to me, but one that everyone knew about. She wanted to move from St-Mathias to Moe's River. With its two thousand people, two grocery stores, two churches, hardware store, and a viable school, Moe's River was a metropolis when compared to St-Mathias.

Madame Arcand wanted Cléophas to sell their tiny shack and the two hundred acres of land it sat on. From the sale of the land they could buy a small house in Moe's River. This was a common practice among the old farming couples, when they had no children or none of their children wanted to continue farming. In Moe's River she could visit and be visited by other older people, attend the Golden Age Club, and not be stuck all day looking across the kitchen table at Cléophas. The only alternative was to go into the bedroom which was completely taken up by the bed. You could understand her position.

Once a week Cléophas and Mathilde drove into Moe's River to go to the bank, buy groceries and visit a few friends. He had no car. For a car he used a tractor on which he had put a tin roof and a small second seat. The sight of the two of them tearing down the road from St-Mathias to Moe's River on this contraption was like an illustration from one of those *Uncle Wiggily's* storybooks that were popular when I was a child. The chapter would be called something like "Uncle Wiggily's Automobile." On one of these trips into town, Madame

Arcand was standing in line at the bank and suddenly slipped to the floor and died. Cléophas came into the bank with a bag of groceries, to find his wife lying dead on the floor with a crowd around her.

Speaking of this event Réjean said: "She got her wish—she died in Moe's River."

Cléophas found living without her difficult. He drank more heavily. Within three months of her death, a married daughter convinced him to sell his house and land, and come and live with her in Sherbrooke, a city of sixty thousand people thirty miles away. After a stormy month with her, the daughter put him in an old people's home.

He still phones me about every three months, and I see him at the hospital in Sherbrooke, where I do a weekly emergency shift. After years of visiting him in his shack, where the sense of him as an individual was so strong, it's a shock to see him looking so anonymous among the other patients in the emergency. The smile has that same newborn quality, but it's less frequent. The will to live is gone:

"I'm not going to live out the winter."

"I may not either," I answer.

The contented newborn smile flashes on the skeletal face.

"I get dizzy," Cléophas continues.

"You've been getting dizzy ever since I've known you."

"I know, but it's worse lately. Especially when I bend down or get out of bed or up from a chair."

"It's from a slowing down of your circulation. The blood doesn't quite get up to the brain as it used to. There's some blockage in the arteries of the neck. If you were younger you could have an operation to clean them out. At eighty-five the operation would be too dangerous. The only thing I can tell you is to try and remember to move slowly when you change position. As I always tell you, Cléophas, one of these days I'm going to have to find an honest job."

He smiles for an instant but then continues wearily:

"And my breathing's getting worse every day."

"Let me listen."

Cléophas takes off his jacket and tie and shirt. In St-Mathias, he only wore a tie to funerals. Now that he lives in the city he feels a visit to the doctor warrants one. I take his pulse and blood pressure and listen to his chest. After sixty or seventy years of smoking, Cléophas

has chronic bronchitis. His chest doesn't sound worse than usual, but since Mathilde's death, Cléophas' level of tolerance to discomfort has declined along with his will to live. He already has one medication for his breathing difficulty, but I decide to add another. I don't like adding another drug, but I feel I have to deal with this diminished tolerance.

"I can help you with the breathing. In addition to the pump you're using four times a day, I want you to take a new pill I'm going to give you twice a day. It will make your breathing easier. If you find it upsets your stomach, or makes you feel like your heart is beating too fast, or you feel anything else new and uncomfortable, stop it and call me. It probably won't do anything like that. It will probably only help your breathing. But never take anything that makes you worse, O.K.?"

"O.K., I'll try it." he answers, smiling like a stubbled newborn. "How's the missus?"

"Fine."

"And the boys?"

"Just fine."

"Say hello to the missus for me."

"I will."

"Did that man who bought my place plant a garden?"

"Not yet."

"That's the first time in sixty years there's no garden there. Anyway, I'd better be going. There's a long line of people out there waiting to see you, and most of them look sicker than me." He begins to dress, stops and turns to me: "You work too hard, you know that?"

"I'm O.K. I like my work."

"I know you like it. But you still have to take care of yourself. You have a young family. No one's going to take care of them if something happens to you."

"I'm O.K. Honest. Give me a call and let me know how the pills work."

Castonguay's plow thumps and scrapes around the curve. That means it's six o'clock. An hour has passed since I began writing about Réjean, René Cyr, Madame Arcand and Cléophas. I love to hear the thump of that plow. It always means there's still an hour left for me to work on my journal. Castonguay has the contract for cleaning the roads in this part of the country. He has a fleet of about a dozen enormous plows, snowblowers and scrapers.

Our house is far from the road so I never see his face on this first early morning trip, but we often pass each other on other trips later in the day. From the giant size of his trucks and plows, I'd always imagined him as a huge and powerful man. I was surprised one day when he came as a patient, to find that he's tiny and frail and wears thick-soled shoes to give him more height.

For me the clang of Castonguay's plow every winter morning at six is like the bell on a channel marker at sea. If I'm up to hear it, and working on my journal, it means I'm on course. I look out the window after the sound. There's a cloud of snow spraying up from where he clattered by. It blends with the tail end of a snowstorm winding down out there.

The sound of the plow rattling down the road gradually fades away. Once again the only sound I hear is the wind sweeping across the hills and buffeting our house. The house is on top of a hill and the land runs down to a river valley. We're exposed to the wind on all sides. The house often shakes in the heavy winds as if it were about to take off down the hill, just as the pages of a patient's medical file did one day, as I was getting out of the car after a house call.

I look out on the snowflakes tossing in the waning storm, and think of the blizzard of people I've met while working as a doctor. Ten years now. A storm of people. Each person like a snowflake in that storm. Each one weaving his way among the others. There's an illusion of strength in the storm. Only an illusion, because in the summer, when I sit here writing my journal early in the morning, there's no snow or howling wind. The sounds I hear are birds calling, cattle bellowing and crickets buzzing. Unless it's a cloudy day, there's an early morning light at the open window and dew from the fields in the air. Winter and that blizzard might never have existed, nor that storm of people, nor me their observer.

But from eight in the morning on, that storm of people will be weaving their way in and out of the office, wanting something for a cough, or the sewing up of a cut, or wanting me to deliver their baby, or arrange for an abortion, or wanting a cure for dizziness, or a refuge from their obsessions, or relief from chest pain, or documentation of their bruises from a police beating, or wanting the strength to cope with an alcoholic husband or a senile parent.

As I get older the storm will thin out, and I'll be left with patients who've aged along with me, who will continue to see me for minor ailments, and go to younger doctors when they're really sick. There's an older doctor not far from me whose telephone number is similar to mine. It's the same digits in a different order. Often people call thinking they're speaking to him, even after I've said my name in answering:

"Listen, George," they say, "my right knee can use a shot of that stuff. And maybe the left one also. I'll be down there in twenty minutes."

That's ahead for me when the storm thins out. But now I'm thirty-nine and the blizzard of people weaves on. For the public I'm at the height of my powers. Old enough to be regarded as experienced, yet young enough to be current in my knowledge. I'm not impressed by this present loyalty. It's about as trustworthy as the attention focused on a steer when he's ripe for slaughter. Like him, I just happen to be maximally useful at this time.

Thirty-nine years old. The practice of medicine is a patchwork of science and showmanship I've been at ten years now. With all its limitations, within the last two or three years I've come to feel comfortable in it. Not complacent. I know I will continually need to go on learning. But comfortable, in that I don't experience the terror that I knew quite frequently for the first year or two after graduation from medical school.

I mean the kind of terror the intern knows on his first night on call, when he wakes to the phone ringing by his bed in the intern's residence, and it's one of the nurses from one of the wards speaking to him, and yet to no one in particular, in a rapid monologue of logarithmically expanding disaster, which seems to have begun sometime before he picked up the phone and will continue on after he puts the phone down:

"…Mrs. Mackintosh who's one day post-op from a hysterectomy. Her respiratory rate is thirty-six per minute. Her blood pressure's seventy systolic. The diastolic's inaudible. Her pulse is a hundred and thirty and regular. She's pale, cold and clammy and doesn't respond to questions…"

You don't know Mrs. Mackintosh, and you don't know why she's in shock. As you run down the silent early morning corridors of the hospital, clutching wildly at different diagnostic possibilities, the thought of trying to distinguish one from the other, and trying to keep the patient alive at the same time, leaves you clammy and sweaty and breathing rapidly yourself, and you wonder how they can call a kid like you to save this woman near death, and you wish they'd call a real doctor, and that you were still sleeping and this were all a dream.

But it isn't a dream, and you muddle through an initial assessment of Mrs. Mackintosh, and quickly call the junior resident to help you. Residents are trainees at various levels beyond internship. Much to the intern's relief, they also sleep in the hospital. If the junior resident needs help he calls the senior resident. If the senior needs help he calls the chief resident, who sleeps at home but will come in if needed. The final resource in the system is the staff doctor, who is also sleeping at home and will come in if needed. After watching the junior resident with this patient, you learn enough so that the next time you're called by a nurse about a patient in shock, you can at least keep your head enough to respond to her monotone of disaster with an appropriately reassuring barrage of orders for her to fulfill while you're on the way:

"Give her one hundred percent oxygen by mask at six litres per minute. Lower the head of the bed. Put in an intravenous line with an eighteen needle. Run in a litre of normal saline. Get a complete blood count, electrolytes and crossmatch her for four units of whole blood. Call the blood gas technician. I'll be there the same time as her…"

You've learned that you have an obligation to be reassuring even if you don't feel reassured yourself. You come to understand that all the nurses expect from you is that you know the basic steps which are similar for almost all emergencies, and keep your uncertainty to yourself until you can share it with someone who knows more than you do.

Aside from the patients like Mrs. Mackintosh who are comatose, most encounters with patients demand both technical skill and a psychologically adept application of that skill. With each experience, a perceptive doctor develops an increasingly honed capacity to perceive the emotional factors at work in illness, and to deal with them in treatment. These same factors must be considered in relating to the patient's family or friends, and all the other people who may be involved in the patient's care, including other doctors, nurses, and technicians. It all becomes very complex and interwoven; that's what I mean by patchwork of science and showmanship.

The doctor who has best achieved that kind of balance is Martin, a West Indian friend of mine. He's a pediatrician who did his training in Montreal and is now living in Kenya. I met him while I was a medical student. My wife Lenore was a technician in the respiratory function laboratory at the Children's Hospital where she and Martin had become friends. He was the chief resident at the time. Residency is generally exhausting; a resident is usually an exploited apprentice. Martin's hiding place was Lenore's corner of the respiratory function lab. Sometimes he would just come to talk, and at other times he would close the door, stretch out on an examination table, and catch up on sleep.

A resident's pay is inadequate for a family and Martin had five children. Even though his wife was a nurse who worked part-time, they were always having to borrow money against the day he would be a practicing pediatrician. As chief resident, Martin was on call at the hospital every second night. On the alternate nights, he often took one of several moonlighting jobs in clinics and emergency rooms around the city to try and diminish his increasing debt.

One of these jobs was substituting on house calls for the staff pediatricians. This was before medicare and payment of the doctor's fee by the government, which we now have in Canada. These were the staff doctors' private patients — they were generally children from wealthy families who lived in exclusive neighbourhoods. Martin used to take me with him on these calls. The patients were stunned to find a bearded, black doctor at the door in place of their familiar, elegant pediatrician. It was equally unsettling that the new black doctor had brought along a long-haired young man whom he introduced as a medical student.

Martin loves children. Watching him with children was mesmerizing. Children who were old enough picked up on the true interest in them and appreciation for them that Martin conveyed. No matter how wary or hostile the parents felt toward this new doctor, they were awed by the powerful interaction between him and their child. That wasn't showmanship. That was genuine love and respect for children. The showmanship was in Martin's style in relating to the parents. When Martin had examined the child he would turn to the parents, "I'll tell you what's wrong with your child."

The parents would lean forward expectantly while Martin paused to put his equipment back in his bag. The bag closed, he would once again turn to them and solemnly say: "He has a cold." He would pause and continue: "I'll tell you in a moment what to do about it."

Then he would disappear into a bathroom to wash his hands. He would come out and explain that though the child was certainly uncomfortable, that it wasn't a serious illness, and that antibiotics would be both unnecessary and useless. Knowing the parent might call another doctor immediately after he left if he prescribed nothing, he would prescribe a decongestant, which we both knew was probably useless and probably harmless. He would phone the pharmacy and order the decongestant syrup as carefully and majestically as if it were a cardiac drug for a patient in heart failure. There's not too much you can do for a cold. But you have to recognize patients' needs in the face of illness. By being absolutely scientific you may just add to their anxiety.

There were usually about ten of these house calls to make. We would finish by about midnight and head for a drink at Rockhead's Paradise Café. Rockhead's was a thriving bar in Montreal's oldest black community. It was where Martin went to relax. Rockhead was a wily, aging, yet ageless West Indian who made a fuss about Martin each time we entered. Rockhead was proud of this young man from the Islands who was doing well as a doctor here in Montreal.

When we got back to his house, Martin would proudly spread the cash he'd earned on the living room floor to count it, and show it to his wife. She was inevitably still folding the wash or ironing. I imagine she probably resented him going for a drink when he could have been helping her fold the clothes. But that's marriage, and that's a whole other world. This journal is about medicine. I don't have the courage to write about marriage.

Another great performer was a native medicine man I met when I was working as a doctor on a Dogrib Indian reservation in the Northwest Territories called Fort Collins. A patient named Rick Whalen had become a friend. His father was a medicine man and Rick had set up a meeting at my request. I had told Rick I was interested in meeting with the medicine men and learning from them. About two months after I had discussed the possibility with Rick, he appeared one night at my door: "My father says tonight would be a good time to meet," Rick said.

Rick's father, Emile, was a small, wiry, taciturn man in his fifties. If he spoke English, he chose not to speak it that night. He nodded a greeting to me as we entered. Anything else he said to me that night was in Dogrib with Rick interpreting. For the first hour of the visit, we sat staring into an oil drum fire. I had only been in Fort Collins for a few months, but I had already spent many hours staring into oil drum fires. It was the favourite pastime. Rick spoke about his plans to teach me how to set rabbit snares. Rick's mother sat on the floor playing cards with a younger child. Some meat was cooking slowly on a corner on the fire. Every ten or fifteen minutes she would reach over to the fire and move the meat slightly.

One thing I did understand from previous hours of staring into fires was that there was no demand for me to introduce myself. There was no interest in my past history, or my origins, or what brought me to Fort Collins. It was clear what I was: the new doctor. If I were a good doctor this would become evident, and if I were a bad one it would also become evident. That's all that really interested them.

As usual it was forty below zero and the wind was howling. Because of the cold nobody takes off their coat when they visit. It's not because the houses are cold. People either had shacks like Emile's which were well heated with oil drum fires, or government built houses with adequate oil heating. The vivid memory of the unbelievable cold you just left makes it reasonable to sit in these warm houses in a fur-lined parka. You want to store up excess warmth before you face that cold again.

Rick was in his early twenties. I'd met him the first night I was in Fort Collins. It was early in September and we'd already had a large snowstorm. I had run one of the medical cars into a ditch. Rick had happened to pass by at that moment and helped me pull it out. I gave him a few dollars for helping. Later at about five in the morning, I was called to the hospital to see two people injured in a car accident. Rick was one of them. He had a long, deep gash of about seven inches running down the front of his lower leg. As I was approaching the hospital he was trying to leave. A nurse was trailing behind him trying to convince him to stay. Rick was drunk. The reason he was leaving was because the nurses were speaking in French to one another.

"If you can't talk Indian, at least talk English!" Rick lamented drunkenly to the nurse, "But why French?"

The reason the nurses spoke French to one another was because they were French nursing nuns who came from Montreal. I explained to him that it was as natural for them to talk French to each other as it was for him and other Dogrib Indians to talk in Dogrib to one another. He came back into the hospital with me and I examined his wound. I did an X-ray of his lower leg to make sure there was no underlying fracture. The X-ray came out over-exposed. Rick resisted taking another one.

At this point I used some of the Dogrib words I had learned. I usually worked with an interpreter, but had been studying the language to be able to handle as much as I could on my own. What I wanted to say to Rick was, if it were my leg, I would want the X-ray repeated. I knew the Dogrib word for leg was "*zah*", and that putting "*ned*" before it as a prefix made it "your leg", and "*zed*" before it made it "my leg". I pointed to his leg, and then my leg, and said:

"*Nedzah zedzah.*"

Your leg is my leg.

Rick smiled and drawled:

"O.K., Doc. In that case you better take another picture."

There was no fracture. I showed him the X-ray. Wherever possible I like sharing the patients' X-ray film with them. It shows the patient you recognize you're dealing with their body, and that you realize they went through a procedure in having an X-ray. For those two reasons alone it seems fitting to share the result with them.

After about an hour of staring into the fire, Rick's father suddenly turned to me and spoke in Dogrib with Rick interpreting:

"When I was young," he said, "my father told me many secrets."

He turned away from me and went back looking into the fire. I waited intently for more. But that was all he said.

About an hour later a man carrying a caribou skin came to the door. He was a patient coming to see Emile. The caribou skin was the fee for Emile's services. Emile took him into the bedroom which was the only other room in the shack.

The Dogrib medicine men work with two main tools, herbs and dream treatment. They use herbs for physical illnesses and dream treatment for psychological problems. In dream treatment the patient comes in the evening and tells the medicine man his problem. The patient leaves and returns in the morning. During the night if all goes well, the medicine man has a dream, in which the solution to the problem becomes evident. If no solution appears in his dream, the medicine man returns the patient's payment to him and tells him to go elsewhere for his answer.

Emile and the patient emerged from the bedroom two minutes later. The patient was still carrying the caribou skin. The patient looked puzzled and downfallen. Emile showed him to the door. After about another ten minutes of staring in the fire, Emile turned to me and spoke. Rick translated:

"Rick will bring you again."

I can take a hint. Apparently my first lesson in native medicine was over. Since my coat was already on I could leave immediately.

The next morning at the clinic I discovered the first lesson was only beginning. My first patient was the man I'd seen last night at Emile's house. He had no caribou skin with him this time, but he did have the same puzzled and defeated expression.

The man spoke no English. I worked with an interpreter. The patient was from one of the outlying settlements. He had travelled hundreds of miles by dogsled to see Emile. The problem was headaches. He had seen Emile three years ago and had been given a satisfactory solution for the problem. The headaches had disappeared. But they had recently reappeared when he had stopped following Emile's advice, "Emile told me I was a damn fool," the patient said dejectedly. "He said he'd told me what to do three years ago, that he had no more time to waste on me, and that I should go and see you."

Before seeing Emile three years ago the patient was having severe headaches several times a month for about a year. In the dream Emile saw the patient dragging a slain moose through his settlement. This was humiliating for the dead moose. Everyone could see who he was. It was more proper to cut off the dead moose's head outside the settlement, and bring it in wrapped, so that the slain moose remained anonymous. Because of his lack of consideration, the angry spirit of the dead moose was entering his head and giving him headaches. In future, were he to cut off the moose's head before entering the settlement, and show the spirit of the angry moose he had learned a lesson, his headaches would cease.

He had followed these instructions faithfully for three years and never had a headache. A month ago he had gotten drunk after killing a moose. In drunken bravado, he figured that the silly curse had probably worn off, and dragged the animal through the settlement with its head on. The next day he had a stupendous headache, and had been having them frequently since.

I sorted through my bag of tricks, knowing in some way I had to match Emile. Even after a relatively short time of working as a doctor among native people, I knew that the classical, detailed medical history which is so assuring to most white patients, is detrimental with native patients. Generally with white people when you are taking a medical history, if you ask a lot of questions they find it reassuring. They feel you are considering many possibilities and not leaping to a diagnosis. Look at all those questions! Look at all the possibilities he's considering. He really knows his stuff. He's considering all the options. Look at all the time he's taking. He's really interested in my problem. Native people on the other hand are used to the intuitive diagnostic style of the native medicine man. The more questions you ask the more it makes them feel that you are floundering. Why is the doctor asking so many questions? He doesn't know what I have! As the number of questions increase, so does the patient's panic. Soon all he wants is to escape from you as soon as possible.

Not squandering my few permissable questions, I satisfied myself that his headaches were not due to a brain tumour or another disease. I felt confident they were tension headaches. The theory for these kind of headaches is that tension causes excess contraction of the scalp muscles, which in turn causes pain. I proceeded to the physical examination and lavished attention on the neurological exam. The nervous system is the most reasonable system to concentrate on when the problem is one of headache, but I also knew it had relevant magical appeal. I solemnly closed the lights in the office, and peered into the back of his eyes with my ophthalmoscope. The optic nerve ending, which is visible as a white disc at the back of the eye, is actually an extension of the brain. The increase of pressure in the brain caused by a brain tumour can cause the optic nerve and disc to swell. His optic discs were normal. I dramatically opened the lights again, and had him follow the motion of my weaving finger to check his eye movements. I had him close his eyes and stand with his hands in front of him, and tested his ability to withstand my gently trying to push him over. These are all relevant and legitimate tests, but done with flourish they can have magical appeal.

His complete examination was normal. Ordinarily, at this point, I would have explained to him that he had tension headaches and told him how I would treat them. But compared to the medicine man's dream treatment, it all would have been too quick. I needed a ritual diagnostic interval similar in time and mystique to the medicine man's overnight dream. Instead of wrapping up the case at this point as I normally would have, I turned to him and said: "I know what's wrong with you."

I paused and reached for an X-ray requisition and began to fill it out. The pause, of course, was a copy of Martin's pausing to put away his stethoscope after saying: "I'll tell you what's wrong with your child." At moments like this Martin is always with me.

"It's not serious and I can definitely help you," I said as I continued to fill the requisition, "but I need to have an X-ray of your head for me to know for sure that I'm right."

I didn't need an X-ray. I knew it would be normal. But it was the perfect substitute for the medicine man's overnight dream. We had an old X-ray machine in our hospital that we used for limbs and chests and abdomens, but a reliable skull X-ray was beyond our scope. He would have to be driven a hundred miles to the hospital in Yellowknife to have the skull film. He left the next morning at six a.m. in the station wagon, with several other patients being sent to Yellowknife for diagnostic tests or admission to hospital. In winter the trip is in total darkness at forty below zero on treacherously icy roads.

In Yellowknife he would no doubt sit for several hours in the X-ray department before he was led to the X-ray table. The massive nozzle of the X-ray camera would be glided into focus on his head. The technicians would tell him: "Don't move!"

He wouldn't understand their words, but their tone would be authoritative and impressive. The camera would whine and click thera-peutically. They would lead him back to the waiting room, and even-tually give him the X-ray films and a radiologist's report to return to me. Usually they only send the report, but in this case I had asked for the films. I wanted to show them to the patient on his return.

The station wagon arrived home at ten-thirty at night. It was now fifty-five below zero and stormy. It had been a harrowing drive. So much the better. I ushered the patient into my office and asked an-other patient who spoke English to remain behind to translate. I was pleased to see the headache patient no longer looked dejected. He looked like a dazed initiate in a religious ceremony. I solemnly took the radiologist's report from him. I opened it ceremoniously and read it to myself:

"Normal skull."

I closed the office lights and flipped the films onto a reviewing screen. The patient's own skull peered back at him from its empty sockets. The patient was in a trance. I flipped on the lights.

"It's just what I thought" I said, as I peered intensely into the nor-mal skull film. "When you get nervous or upset the muscles in your scalp become tight." I clenched my fists to indicate what I meant by tight. "That causes the headache."

I paused to take the skull films off the screen and put them back into their envelope. Pauses are important. I turned on the lights and sat down at my desk. I slowly and deliberately reached for a prescrip-tion pad.

"Here's what we're going to do about it," I continued. "First, when you get these headaches you shouldn't be frightened by them anymore. Now you know why you're getting them. Try figure out why you're nervous or upset, and try to do something about it. From that alone it may go away. If it doesn't, you can take one of these pills I'm going to give you."

The translator turned to him and said everything I said in about six Dogrib words. He was either very articulate or very tired.

I gave him a medication used for tension headaches and migraine. It's a mixture of aspirin with a small dose of phenobarb. Some caffeine is added to overcome any drowsiness the phenobarb may cause. I know they're effective because I've taken them myself for migraine. In my case I've found they not only take away the headache, but they also have a euphoric effect. I said at the beginning of this journal that I love my work. After one or two of those pills, I really love it.

In his case, along with the aspirin, phenobarb and caffeine, there would always be the memory of a trek to Yellowknife for a skull X-ray, and a doctor peering intently into a glowing picture of his skeletal head, and a doctor dancing around him in a darkened room, waving his arms and peering into his eyes with an intense light. I gave him a few pills and a prescription for several repeats. In outlying settlements, like the one he lived in, there was usually someone who was the custodian of a supply of medication. They were called lay dispensers. They received a course in basic first aid and rudimentary pharmacology. They are somewhat like the "barefoot doctors" of Communist China, except that nobody goes barefoot most of year in the Canadian North.

He left with the pills. About a year later I received a letter from the lay dispenser in his settlement. He wanted some more of the pills for the patient. The letter said they were working very well: the patient only had to use them three times. The headache had stopped within a few minutes after taking them. The dispenser was writing for more because I hadn't written an expiry date on the bottle, and he wondered if they were still good.

The pills worked. They weren't matching Emile Whalen's three year headache free record as yet. But perhaps as they continued to work effectively, the whole issue of headache would be less threatening, and just fall out of the patient's life for good. In a short time the frequency of the headaches was already much less. At this rate we might be moving towards their disappearance.

I waited for my next formal meeting with Emile. There were none for the present. But there were frequent patient referrals. These were the lessons for now.

Fort Collins

Outlaw Status

FORT COLLINS, a Dogrib Indian settlement in the Northwest Territories, is a sub-Arctic favella of wooden shacks clinging to the rocky windswept shore of Great Slave Lake. Seen from an airplane it looks as if the next blast of the almost perpetually blowing wind will buffet the village into the lake.

The Dogribs live and hunt between Great Slave Lake and Great Bear Lake, which is two hundred and fifty miles further north. Geographers call the area a zone of "stunted tree growth". The trees are short, sparsely branched and grow farther apart than trees in southern Canada. Further north the stunted trees fade out, and the moss covered terrain called the Barren Ground leads up to the true Arctic. The land is covered in snow three quarters of the year. In mid-winter the temperature ranges between thirty and fifty degrees below zero. By Christmas time there are only a few hours of daylight. During those few hours on looking up at the sky at a random moment, it's hard to decide if the sun is going up or coming down.

Of the two thousand Dogribs, about sixteen hundred live in Fort Collins. The remaining four hundred live in three small satellite settlements within a few hundred miles radius of Fort Collins. There are no roads connecting the three outlying settlements to Fort Collins or to each other. They can only be reached by airplane, by dog team or snowmobile in winter, or by canoe on a system of rivers, lakes and portages in summer.

The name Dogrib is derived from the tribe's belief that the Great Spirit created the First Man out of the rib of a Dog. Sound familiar? They believe they were the first men. Maybe they were. The name Fort Collins was conferred on this Indian village by white men in honour of a white man. Sir Richard Collins was a nineteenth century Hudson's Bay Company official. The first visit of a doctor to Fort Collins was made at the turn of the century. There was no road to Fort Collins at the time. The doctor came by boat travelling up Great Slave Lake. He is still remembered for the lethal influenza epidemic that immediately followed his visit.

The Dogribs call Fort Collins *Batesokon*, which in Dogrib means

"Downtown," so defining its relation to the three outlying settlements. The mining town of Yellowknife, one hundred miles away, the administrative center of the white appointed territorial government, they call *Sambake*. *Samba* means money. *Ke* means "where it is."

Fort Collins is made up of about three hundred shacks. Outside of at least two thirds of them is a pen made of logs for keeping a family's sled dogs chained to stakes. The tops of these logs are chopped to a point. In winter the Dogribs fish through the ice on Great Slave Lake, and on returning home they impale the freshly caught fish on the points of the logs. At forty below zero the fish freeze onto the log in a few hours. The Dogribs call these frozen fish stickfish. That's fishsticks backwards. All winter they simply break the fish off the poles and feed them to the dogs.

Deep freezing is easy in Fort Collins. On the drive from Yellowknife, the Dogribs often stop to shoot ptarmigan, which are white birds similar to partridges. They throw them in the trunks of their cars, and on arriving back home in Fort Collins two hours later, find them deep frozen. Likewise, almost deep frozen was a drunk who had fallen in a stupor outside the pool-hall. Among the Dogribs a tribal decree prohibits drinking alcohol. The Dogribs had walked by him and left him there. This man had been fool enough to ignore the decree. He could bear the consequences. It was the white officers of the RCMP, or Royal Canadian Mounted Police, who brought him to the hospital before he froze to death. The code for survival at forty below zero has no frills.

Calculate two hundred shacks having an average of about eight dogs chained outside each one. You can then see why there was almost always the sound of dogs barking in Fort Collins. The Dogribs maintained they would howl loudest when someone was dying. Walking at night from our house to the hospital, under frozen skies crammed with stars and pulsating with the Northern Lights, I would involuntarily gauge the volume of the dogs' howling. If it seemed louder, I would do a mental ward rounds of the hospitalized patients, wondering where I might have gone wrong.

Another sound that was always present in Fort Collins was the wind. Each morning from our window, we could gauge the wind velocity by the volume and intensity of the flapping of a Canadian flag in front of the town hall. The rest of the day the sound of the wind was always with you: strong in your ears as you walked outside struggling in it, or softer and moaning as you went about your work inside.

The third perpetual sound by day, in addition to the dogs and the wind, was the cry of the northern ravens. They are large black scavenging birds somewhere between the size of overgrown crows and small vultures. They shriek into the wind as they pick their way through bits of frozen garbage. They have no fear of humans. With a sense of irony I admired, the local teenage rock group called themselves the Ravens. The teenagers for the most part looked like bikers without motorcycles. Occasionally, they would succeed in getting some old car to run for a few hours, and scrape together enough money to head for Yellowknife. But generally there wasn't much in the way of action. Rock music on records and tapes, and on the radio from Yellowknife, kept them in loose touch with North American teenage culture, but without television as a guide, the assimilation was erratic.

Take for example the adolescence of Johnny Swallow, the hospital driver and my interpreter. Johnny was now in his early twenties, but he was still living out the consequences of an ambivalent and partial absorption of the ways of the outside world. At eighteen he had been chosen to receive a government grant to go south to Vancouver, to learn how to build fibreglass boats. Some bureaucrats in Indian Affairs, who had never been to Fort Collins, decided that fiberglass canoes would be an improvement over whatever kind of canoes the Dogribs made. There was vague talk of creating a fibreglass canoe factory in Fort Collins. Johnny took the training in Vancouver for two years. The factory never materialized. When he finished his training there was no way to apply it in Fort Collins. He was offered a well paying job in Vancouver by the company who had trained him. He refused it and returned to Fort Collins with a suede jacket and tapered jeans, and has worn both ever since, no matter how cold it gets. At about forty below he'll wear a parka over the jacket.

Johnny refused the job in Vancouver because, for him, Fort Collins with its two hundred shacks and howling dogs, is home and the centre of the universe. Johnny was very handsome. He was tall, slim and broad shouldered. There was vague talk of a white girl in Vancouver who had jilted him, and left him in a state of relative mourning ever since. Indians like nicknames. Everyone in Fort Collins had one. Because of his height, Johnny was called "Stringbean".

I had learned from one of the priests that my nickname was "The Bushy-Haired Doctor". This I hoped was not to be confused with the "bushmen" or *nagaan* who were evil men-demons with bushy hair and long, dirty nails who would kill hunters lost in the woods. My wife Lenore, who laughs a lot, was called "Crazy Laughing Lady."

I was called one midnight to see an old couple in their shack after they had been robbed. The old man had been struck on the head. He was Ronnie Mackenzie, the former chief of the tribe, who had retired because of failing health. He was not seriously injured. There were a lot of people milling around the shack.

I examined the old man. All he needed were some cold compresses for a slight bruise. On the way out I asked one of the men if it was known who had done it: "Johnny Swallow," came the reply.

"Johnny?" I questionned incredulously.

"Yes," the man answered assuredly. "The old chief says when he asked who was knocking, the person outside said 'Stringbean.'"

It was a crude frame-up. As the medical driver Johnny had frequently taken the ailing Ronnie to and from the hospital. The thief knew this. He had used this association as a way to enter easily. The old chief might think the doctor had sent for him. Ronnie opened the door without a moment's hesitation. The thief rushed in, knocked him on the head, shoved his wife aside, rifled through the shack for money, found it and ran off. In the dark, Ronnie had never really seen who it was.

The next day the RCMP officers had the real thief. He was a well-known alcoholic who had stolen the money to buy liquor. I knew him from another episode. Once in a drunken rage he had run over his pregnant wife with a snowmobile. We had attempted to have him prosecuted at that time, but the wife had refused to press charges.

In our work together, Johnny took a stance toward me that always reminded me of the people who let the stuporous drunk lie freezing to death outside the poolhall. He usually let me make mistakes without commenting on them. One exception was the time I was packing drugs to take with me on my first clinic in one of the outlying settlements. As I started to close up the bag, Johnny blurted out: "Aren't you going to bring along some of the rub for rheumatism?"

He took some menthol and camphor muscle rub from the drug shelf and brought it to me. He was very uncomfortable in offering advice. He wished this wasn't happening. He didn't look at me as he spoke: "The old people like the rub," he said.

Many of the old people living in the bush had arthritis. Some of them lived in tents despite frequent spells of fifty and sixty below zero temperatures. For them the warmth and comfort found in menthol and camphor balms was the only use they could see in the doctor and his monthly flight in for a clinic. I had rarely prescribed muscle rub in southern Canada. It had never occurred to me to put it in the critical supply of drugs to be taken on an airplane flight with severe cargo limits. But to have arrived without it would have been a clear statement of incompetence that Johnny could not bear witnessing. He had borne the discomfort of giving me advice, rather than the shame that would have resulted for both of us had he let me go unwarned. But he had hated doing it. After he had seen me place the tubes of muscle rub in the bag, he went off in a corner to have a smoke, and recuperate from the whole encounter.

One road circled Fort Collins and continued on a desolate one hundred miles along Great Slave Lake to Yellowknife. Most of the year the road was as icy as a bobsled run. If it were nightime or bad weather with few people out, slipping off the road on a deserted stretch between Fort Collins and Yellowknife could mean freezing to death before someone passed who could help to get the car back on the road.

During the first few days at Fort Collins, I was called out to pronounce two truck drivers dead after their oil tanker had slipped off the road, struck a tree and exploded. It had happened about thirty miles from the village. I was driven there in the ambulance with Father Raynaud, one of the priests in the settlement. I was very tired. I had delivered a baby the night before, and had gone without much sleep the night previous to that one tending two very sick patients in the hospital. Rather than sit up in front with the ambulance driver and Father Raynaud, I lay down in the stretcher in the back and tried to sleep. I could tell my lying down in the stretcher annoyed Father Raynaud. He would have liked me, as a member of the local white gentry, to suffer my fatigue with dignity. Trying to rest in public was vulgar.

Father Raynaud was one of two priests in Fort Collins; he lived in the main settlement. The other priest rotated living in the three outlying settlements. Father Raynaud was an adept politician; he was the director of the hospital and advisor to the schoolboard. The hospital had originally been founded as a mission by an order of French nuns from Montreal. Over the years the Canadian Government had stepped in to help. The way it stood at present was that I was an employee of the government. The clinic and office in which I worked in the hospital was the financial responsibility of the government. The moment the patient was hospitalized he was a ward of the church. The five nurses in the hospital were nuns.

The schoolboard was nominally Dogrib, but Father Raynaud ran it in his capacity as an advisor. His political power was enhanced by a close friendship with the government appointed manager of the town council, who in effect functioned as a colonial administrator for the Canadian government in the settlement. Father Raynaud and this government-appointed administrator ruled the settlement. The chief was merely a figurehead. Any project the chief might want to undertake required government money. The government acted on the advice of the manager of the town council, who was a white civil servant imported from southern Canada. From behind a screen of what was called native self-determination, Father Raynaud and the town manager exercised absolute power. It was a medieval fusion of church and state. It was a power base backed by a secular army of government bureaucrats and government supported private industry. As my stay evolved I was naive enough to challenge their power. My opposition to them proved no threat at all. It was merely the occasion for a militia drill.

Before I met Father Raynaud and the town manager, I used to think that a song Johnny Cash sings about shooting someone "just to see them die" was too violent. After meeting them I didn't think so. But I look upon them fondly now as my first instructors in the karate of politics. First lesson: How strong the provider! How large the biceps of he who furnishes food and warmth. Their power is based on people who depend on their power. It's a self-perpetuating cycle difficult to interrupt. I had no idea how difficult.

They were such good teachers of the karate of politics, that I learned the second lesson simultaneously with the first: just when you're expecting a pat on the back, you'll be dealt a blow on the back of the neck. Since then I've never stopped learning. The number of lessons is infinite. The black belt? Forever receding: like the clown's hat, continuously kicked ahead by his own toe as he bends to pick it up.

We arrived at the exploded oil truck. The two men in it had been burned to death. Both bodies were so charred it looked as if one touch would render them to ashes. I signed a police report and quickly returned to the warmth of the ambulance and the joy of laying down on the luxurious stretcher. Father Raynaud stayed around outside another ten minutes after he said the last rites, doing nothing but proving he could tolerate cold better than I could.

The ambulance headed back to the settlement. The whine of the tires on the ice drowned out the conversation up front between Father Raynaud and the ambulance driver. The driver was a white school teacher who drove the ambulance on a volunteer basis. He was also irritated by my laying on the stretcher, and made a few caustic remarks about it. They could both go to hell. The priest and his parishioner. I lay there enjoying the first real peace I'd had since I'd arrived in Fort Collins. It was the first time I'd been inaccessible since I'd arrived. In rural situations that feeling is rare for a doctor. You live right by your work. Whether at the clinic or in your house, you're always accessible. Here I was hurtling along in the back of the ambulance completely out of reach. I felt like a teenager again.

I had felt especially tense in the first weeks at finding myself the only doctor around. I must have been showing the strain because someone left some graffiti on the wall of the clinic which read:

"The new doctor never smiles."

The message scrawled on the wall put me at ease. I could stop trying to pretend I was invincible. There were more experienced doctors who knew more than me. But they weren't here. I was; and I could only do my best. That whole day I smiled to myself whenever

I thought of the message. It felt good that some unknown person out there had cared enough to tell me to look after myself.

I'd come to Fort Collins for two main reasons. One was because they needed a doctor. I wanted to work where I felt needed. The second was because I wanted to learn what native people knew about living in North America. Both my father and mother were Russian Jews who had come to Canada in their childhood. Their families had left their villages in Russia at the turn of the century. They had crossed the North Atlantic and disembarked at the city of Montreal on the St. Lawrence river as some of their relatives had done earlier, and had instructed them to do. The native people had also come to Canada from Russia. They had come much earlier and to the western end of Canada when there had been a connection by land across the Bering Strait. The native people came here many thousands of years before my people. I thought I'd see what they knew about the place.

The Arctic ravens were unmoved by my quest for this primal knowledge. They'd been picking through the frozen garbage a long time before I'd gotten here, and would still be picking at it a long time after I'd left. At bad moments their mocking cry mingled with the howling of the dogs and the moaning of the wind would rise in my ears like a weary chorus in a Greek drama, reminding me that my fate was largely the consequence of my folly. The Dogribs with their language I didn't understand were a pantomime element in the same drama: poker-faced mummers who had seen many doctors passing through, and almost never staying more than a year. Here comes another. The fact that I was there because I felt there was an essential need to fill medically, and was making about one fifth the amount of money I could make in southern Canada, was clear to nobody but me. The assumption was that I was here because I would be paid more than in the south, or worse—that I was too inexperienced to get a good job in the south. In a setting with a history marked by several hundred years of massacre and treachery, sincerity is most often seen as weakness. There's little room for it on the stage. The main characters already have their roles. The white man works at manipulating the native people for his end, while the native people work at manipulating the white man for theirs. Each allows the other to think they are in control, while the real powers are government and industry in southern Canada, who foster the illusion that final control resides in a nation of voters.

In my appearance on stage, there was however, one unusual element that I only became aware of after about six months at Fort Collins. I had a clinic assistant called Anna. She was a combination receptionist, secretary, and stockkeeper. She also worked as an interpreter when Johnny was driving the ambulance. She was a wise person who dealt very well with people. In contrast to Johnny, she was always ready to give me her advice on how to and how not to relate to Dogribs. Her suggestions were always helpful. It was when I was seeing Anna's father as a patient that I was made aware of my special role in Fort Collins. He had come in with his skin red, thickened and burning from head to foot. It was due to a photosensitive skin reaction which occurs because of particularly intense ultraviolet light reflecting off the snow at certain times of the year. Fortunately, it can be cured by a few days of intravenous cortisone. It is mostly seen between January and April. I told him to avoid prolonged exposure to sunlight until September to be safe. I wrote him a note for the welfare department saying that he couldn't work as a trapper or hunter during that period. He came to see me in the clinic not long after his discharge, complaining that he was not receiving welfare. I told him I couldn't imagine why not, but would find out.

Johnny had been interpreting. I asked Anna to come into the room because it involved her family. She explained that her parents were already receiving a welfare payment for her mother who had just had an operation, and was unable to do her usual work in the school kitchen. A family could only get welfare payment for one wage earner. Neither her mother or father had real sickness compensation linked to their jobs. The welfare payment was less than real sickness compensation would have paid. They were finding it difficult.

"Why don't we ask Father Raynaud to help?" I asked Anna. I figured Father Raynaud would do better with the welfare officers than I would. I knew there were two of them: an up-front Dogrib with a whiteman boss. I was new and suspect—if only for that reason. Raynaud knew them well.

"He won't help." Anna answered.

"Why do you say that?" I asked.

"He's a white man," Anna replied bitterly. "White men don't care," she continued.

"What do you mean white men don't care?" I answered angrily. "You see me working here day and night. Is it because I don't care?"

"You're not a white man. You're a Jew." I really laughed. I hadn't imagined Anna or any other Dogrib knew there was such a thing as a Jew. "How did you know I'm Jewish?"

"Father Raynaud told us. He said the Jews killed Christ, but not to hold it against you personally."

"That was generous of him," I said.

That particular attempt by Father Raynaud to alienate me completely backfired. It gave me outlaw status. Being a Jew and a Christ-killer gave me a kind of mystique, and some of the kind of aura surrounding the Dogribs' own black magic medicine men. I'd met one once when he had pneumonia. His name was Louis Watunda. I almost shudder even now as I write his name and wonder if he might curse me for it. Louis Watunda was much feared. You went to him if you wanted someone hexed. The time I'd met him was against his will. It was also against mine. Father Raynaud had dragged me to Louis' shack, even though Louis had said he didn't want the doctor. He was huddled in bed with shaking chills. He was sweating and coughing up bloody sputum. With every cough he lurched with pain. He glowered at me. I guess as a medicine man it was humiliating for him to be treated by the white doctor. But his discomfort prevailed. He allowed himself to be driven to the hospital in the ambulance. He had a good response to intravenous penicillin. By the next day, with Johnny interpreting, he appeared to be a polite, cooperative patient. But I never knew how he felt about the whole episode. I always wondered whether I'd been cursed for my efforts. Nothing has ever turned up beyond the usual ups and downs, so I probably wasn't—unless there's some heavy-duty, delayed-action curse waiting for me somewhere down the line.

Although I may have escaped being hexed by Louis Watunda, I met someone who hadn't. His name was Richard Zoe. In Richard's case there was real heart in the hex, because Louis had cursed him for reasons of his own, and not at someone else's request. Richard had slapped one of Louis' daughters. I don't know what had prompted this rash act, but the net result was he'd slapped her. From that day on Richard had nothing but bad luck. It included a fire in his house and a year in prison. My meeting him was a consequence of his habitual bad luck.

I met Richard when I was on a trip to Yellowknife to visit some patients from Fort Collins, whom I'd admitted to the hospital there. I had arranged to meet Johnny at a restaurant near the hospital at the end of the day. When I got to the restaurant, Johnny was sitting at a table having a beer with a man with a radiant smile and an easy laughter. I sat down and ordered a drink. I knew Johnny wouldn't formally introduce the other man. I find it's not generally what native people do. But being a white man, and used to punctuating situations like this with some kind of introductory ritual, I nodded towards him. He smiled and nodded back.

I got up to go to the men's room and Johnny followed me. I knew he was doing it just to speak to me about the man at our table. I knew what was coming: Johnny was going to ask me if we could drive Richard back to Yellowknife. He tapped me on the shoulder and said: "Doctor, can we drive Richard back to Yellowknife?"

Johnny knew it was against government regulations to give anyone a ride in a government vehicle. The reason was that in case of accident the government would have to pay compensation. Johnny also knew that I would say yes.

"How did he get in?" I asked.

"He came in his own truck. But driving in he hit an Arctic owl and it shattered his windshield. His name's Richard Zoe. Things like that are always happening to him. He was cursed by Louis Watunda. He slapped Louis' daughter, and ever since then he's had nothing but bad luck."

"It doesn't seem to bother him much." I said. "He seems like a pretty happy guy."

"I guess he just lives with it and tries to forget about it."

Johnny knew I was going to say yes. I wasn't that sympathetic to someone who slapped women, but then again he couldn't drive back to Fort Collins without a windshield. And as for the slap, Louis Watunda seemed to be effectively meting out punishment. There seemed no need for me to pile on. Also, he seemed to be Johnny's friend and

4 5

Johnny would feel humiliated if I said no. Johnny knew I was going to say yes, because he had seen me say yes time and again. All these acts of easy-going, affable rule-breaking were being recorded. Not by Johnny but by Father Raynaud, the town manager and the people in their employ. It all caught up with me eventually. Not that I really cared or felt I had done wrong. But it was shocking to see them drag it all out when the time came.

When I was a child, I remember reading in a science book about the fish at the bottom of the sea. As the depth increases, and the sunlight tapers off, vegetation becomes increasingly scarce. For sustenance the fish must devour one another. Their weapons of defence and offence become appropriately heightened. Some fish, for example, have loose-jointed jaws which can expand in an instant to devour fish equal in size to themselves. So it was at times among people in the dark and frozen north.

Johnny, Richard Zoe and I drove home the hundred miles from Yellowknife to Fort Collins. It was fifty-two below zero. Once on a similar night ride, when I had my family with me, the heater of the government car stopped working. We had to drive the rest of the way shivering and fearing the motor might be next to fail. At fifty below zero, if your car stalls, and no one passes by all night, you can freeze to death. Tonight the heater was working. Richard Zoe smiled off into the darkness. I hoped that Louis Watunda would leave him be for the next hundred miles. I found myself smiling.

A Favour for the Chief

ONCE A WEEK I would charter a plane from Yellowknife and fly to one of the outlying settlements to hold a clinic. I would usually decide at the last minute when I was going and which settlement it would be. Late one afternoon I would call a charter company in Yellowknife and arrange for a plane the next morning. There were several telephone extensions in the hospital. Within five minutes after I got off the telephone, someone from the village would knock on the door and say something like: "I hear you're going to Otter Lake. Could you please bring this package to my uncle David Mantla?"

That first person would drop a package in the corner and disappear. This would go on all afternoon, and later at my home that night, and continue on until the last moments of boarding the plane the next morning.

For most people in the village, the main value of the doctor in their life was that he could deliver and pick up packages to and from the outlying settlements. I learned that on my first flight. It was a day in late August. We flew over hundreds of miles of uninterrupted forests and lakes. The clouds above and the airplane itself were reflected in the lakes below. I felt the same feeling of peace and unassailability I had on ambulance trips to Yellowknife: no one could reach me for the moment with a new problem. After an hour or so of flying, at the end of one of those lakes we saw a tiny clump of houses and tents. As we circled for a landing on the lake, people began scurrying out of the houses and tents. They were all assembled on the edge of the pier as we floated up on the plane's pontoons. Everyone was smiling broadly; they were totally elated to see us. As we disembarked, everyone, smiling broadly, ignored us and went for the packages, leaving Johnny and I with more medical equipment and drugs than four people, let alone two, could carry. No one offered to help. We made two trips to the house the clinic was being held in, while everyone concentrated on the distribution of the packages.

The houses in the settlements were generally one room shacks. A blanket was hung from the ceiling to divide the shack into a waiting room and examining room. Usually about twenty patients would wait on one side of the blanket while I examined patients on the other side. There were often one or two patients sick enough to be brought back in the plane with us to be put in the hospital in Fort Collins.

One day, an hour after I had phoned Yellowknife to arrange for a plane for a settlement visit, Johnny told me that the chief of the tribe was out in the waiting room with his interpreter and wanted to see me. He wasn't sick. There was something he wanted to discuss.

I was very proud. I had only been in Fort Collins a few months. The chief wanted to talk about something. I couldn't imagine what it might be, but I was sure it was something about the health of the community in general. Some large issue that he wanted the doctor to play a role in. I thought of coming back home later that day and saying to Lenore: "The chief asked me for his help today."

I knew the chief was largely a front man manipulated by Father Raynaud and the settlement manager, but I put that out of my mind for the moment.

Chief Drybones and his interpreter were seated in my office. They sat in their parkas. I had already learned that it was futile to invite them to take off their coats. It was fifty below zero. We smiled and nodded a greeting to one another. I asked the interpreter: "What is it the chief would like to discuss?"

"He's heard you're going to Otter Lake tomorrow. Is that correct?"

"Yes, that's true. What about it?"

I was starting to feel depressed. I knew what was coming.

"Isadore Chocolate has two caribou legs there he would like to give to the chief. Could you bring them back with you?"

I was completely deflated. Just another package delivery.

"Tell him I could deliver one. Not two. And only if I have no patients to evacuate."

The chief sulked when my answer was translated. He nodded sullenly and left.

The request for two legs was outrageous. Each leg could weigh well over fifty pounds. In terms of cargo space even one was a major demand. I knew where his request for two was coming from. The previous week when I had no patients to transport on a settlement flight, someone at the settlement had asked me to bring a caribou leg back to Fort Collins for someone. The man receiving the leg was on the tribal council. He was a political rival of the chief's. The chief must have heard that the doctor had transported a leg for this rival. The chief was going to show that he was more powerful by having me transport two legs. What I hadn't mentioned to the chief in all this was that if there was going to be room for a leg to be transported, I was hoping to buy one for my own use. The chief had access to many different kinds of tribal business flights. He really didn't need to use the medical plane. He was just doing it as an exercise in political power. Because I had transported a leg for his rival, I would take one for him before one for myself, but two was out of the question.

At Otter Lake the next day it was so cold my ballpoint pen froze. I borrowed a pencil to write notes on the patients' charts. It was a long clinic with many patients to be seen. Two patients had to be evacuated. One was a man in heart failure who needed immediate hospitalization. The second was a child of two with a severe infection in his hip. He had a fever of 104 degrees. He needed surgery immediately. It was probably already too late to avoid some permanent damage in the joint, but it wasn't too late to save it from total destruction. He needed to be flown a thousand miles south to Edmonton where there were pediatric orthopedic surgeons who could best handle his case. I put in an intravenous and began antibiotic treatment which would be continued until his operation.

It was mid-winter and there were only two hours of daylight. As there were no lights on the airplane landing areas, if I didn't finish the clinic before sundown, we would have to sleep over till the next day. When emergency flights had to be made at night, the landing areas were lit up with oil drum fires. The light provided by the oil drum fires was spotty and hazy. It was like landing in some dim smoking plain in hell. They were risky landings and only attempted in extreme medical emergencies.

I managed to finish the clinic with enough daylight time to land at Fort Collins within a few minutes from sundown. As we circled Fort Collins in the waning light, we could see people scurrying out of their shacks and heading for the landing strip to see what packages we had from Otter Lake. We had none. The man in heart failure and the sick baby were the only cargo. At forty below zero, to avoid engine strain, the cargo restrictions were such that even these two extra passengers were excess weight. When the plane landed, Johnny announced to the assembled crowd that there were no packages. The crowd dispersed rapidly, leaving Johnny to handle the medical equipment and supplies by himself. I was carrying the baby. The chief stood about fifty yards from the plane with two other men waiting for his two caribou legs. As I passed him, I explained to one of the men with him, who I knew spoke English, that I had been unable to transport anything because of the two patients I had brought. I explained hurriedly that the child was very ill. Several seconds later, from behind my back, I heard the chief utter the first and only English word I ever heard him speak:

"Liar!" he snarled.

I whipped around. I was angry. I was fed up with the pettiness of the whole thing. A crowd started to collect. I wanted to tell him exactly what I felt, but didn't want to keep the sick child out in the cold. Since he spoke enough English to call me a liar, I now spoke to him directly in English:

"I have a sick baby to take care of. I would like to talk to you alone inside after I do that. It will take about a half hour."

I had a nurse settle the baby into a crib, and phoned down to Edmonton to arrange his transfer for surgery. It was a thousand mile trip. It took at least a half hour to phone to arrange for a flight, a nurse escort, and for transferring of the baby from the airport to the hospital. To my surprise the chief waited the half hour. The bilingual man who had been beside him had waited with him to translate. I wondered how much he needed him. I invited them into my office.

"Why did you call me a liar?" I asked the chief.

The bilingual man translated and promptly returned the chief's reply:

"This is not the first time you've lied to me."

I was stunned, I had never had any previous dealings with him.

"I'm not lying to you now and I've never spoken to you before. I had to transport two sick people. Your people. What's more important to you? Two people or two caribou legs? And when else am I supposed to have lied to you?"

The only answer I received was a silent glower. The silence continued for two or three minutes until the two men rose and left.

I only found out a year later what really happened in that conversation. During that year I came to know the chief's daughter Margaret. She was in her early twenties and had come to me with her two year old who had whooping cough, which can be a long and discouraging illness. After the initial attack, it can linger for months in the form of a persistent cough. The microbe involved is not affected by antibiotics. There is little to do but wait till the infection runs its course. Because of the dramatic and distressing spasms and whoops of coughing, it makes doctors feel uncomfortably helpless. The baby probably wouldn't have gotten the illness if he had been immunized.

But like many Dogrib mothers, Margaret was reluctant to give a needle to a well child, and had never brought him in for any immunization.

Margaret came to see me one day in mid-winter. Her baby had whooping cough now for six weeks and was still coughing. I examined him and did a chest X-ray. There was no secondary pneumonia. I felt uncomfortable but could offer nothing but reassurance, cough syrup and the reminder to use a vaporizer beside his bed. All three of these suggestions, particularly the reassurance, are of little use in the face of overwhelming attacks of spasmodic coughing often followed by vomiting. As she was leaving she asked:

"My dad wants me to take Phillip to Otter Lake. Would that be all right?"

"No. You shouldn't. Not for another month. The temperature is more even in your house in Fort Collins. You can also keep the humidifier going here. There you can't. It's also better to have him nearby, in case, as sometimes happens, he gets another infection on top of the whooping cough."

About a week later, I received a radio call from Otter Lake. It was about Phillip. He was out at Otter Lake and he had gotten worse. His cough was worse and he had a high fever. I ordered a plane from Yellowknife and flew out to Otter Lake. Phillip had pneumonia. I started him on antibiotics and insisted that he return to Fort Collins.

Margaret was unhappy. "Couldn't we stay here?" she grumbled. "My father wants us to stay. The caribou are here now." She sat thinking. It was all too inconvenient. "Alphonse McKenzie says he can cure Phillip's cough", she said.

I knew Alphonse as a patient. That same day I had treated him with an injection of cortisone for bursitis in his shoulder. I hadn't known he was a colleague.

"Why don't you let him?" I asked.

"He wants two caribou skins," Margaret answered.

Caribou skins could be sold to the Hudson Bay store for about five dollars. My flight out cost the government sixteen hundred dollars.

About a year after the caribou leg incident, I approached Margaret and said I needed her help. I explained that her father and I had once had an argument, but a new issue had come up which required our cooperation. I asked her to arrange a meeting and serve as translator.

Government officials intended to close down the hospital and construct one in a new village they were building several miles away. The new village was a mistake. The idea had come from bureaucrats living a thousand miles to the south in Edmonton who had never seen Fort Collins. The mistake was that the new village was miles from the lake.

The Dogribs fished in the lake summer and winter. When the caribou were scarce, fish was the main food. Fish was the staple food for the sled dogs at all times. In the summer a man laid his nets in the morning and returned at dusk to haul in a net full of trout, whitefish and pike. In the winter nets were set through holes in the ice. The lake was the trail's end and beginning for a system of waterways that linked the three outlying settlements to Fort Collins. Airplanes landed on pontoons in the lake in the summer. In the winter the vast stretch of lake was the airplane runway for landing on skis. Beyond these practical considerations, the administrators didn't understand that living with the great lake in view was as essential as breathing to these people. Hearing the wind over the lake, and watching the lines of water birds hovering and turning were sounds and sights that brought order and meaning to each day, each year, each season and each life.

The reason given for changing the location of the settlement was sanitation. It was said that the rock base under the village made construction of a plumbing system impossible. The Dogribs pointed out that the white mining town of Yellowknife a hundred miles down the lake was built on the same rock. The government had already constructed thirty houses in the new village. Even though the rent was nominal, and the houses all had central heating and hot water, hardly any Dogribs had moved there. The only people willing to live there were the white schoolteachers and maintenance staff of the new school the government had built there. Children from Fort Collins were driven by bus every morning to this new school in the empty new village and driven back each night. The government had thought that moving the school to the new village would cause a mass migration of families to live there. No one moved. The government hoped that putting the hospital in the new village would finally convince the Dogribs to move there.

Father Raynaud supported the move. Moving the Dogribs to this suburb without a city would make them more dependent on the church. Cutting them off from their cosmological link to the lake would tame their spirit and allow the church to step in and fill the spiritual void that would result. With the government and the church behind the move, with the school already moved, it seemed almost futile to try and stop it. But I thought I would try.

I told Margaret I had to speak to her father to encourage him to organize a resistance movement. She returned an hour later and said that her father would see me that night.

That night, with Margaret as translator, the chief said he agreed that moving the hospital was unthinkable. He said that the tribe felt that the new village was a threat to their way of life and would result in increasing dependence on the white man. Moving the hospital was completely unacceptable. They had called for a meeting with the government officials from the south who had advocated the move. They were determined to stop it. He said if the government ignored their views, and moved the hospital to the new village, they would burn it down.

Since things were going well, I asked Margaret to ask him why he had called me a liar, and why he had said that I had lied to him even before the caribou leg incident.

"He says he didn't call you a liar," Margaret answered, "and he wants to know why you called him a fool."

"I never called him a fool."

Margaret began to smile and asked: "Who translated?"

"I don't know who he was." I answered. "He was just a man standing near your father."

Still smiling, she repeated the question in Dogrib to her father.

"Isadore Moosenose", he answered and began to smile.

Margaret explained why they were smiling. Isadore Moosenose was a political rival of Chief Drybones. He had been a contender in the election for chief and lost. It was clear that Isadore had taken my invitation to serve as translator to augment the quarrel between the chief and the doctor.

In the long run, far from burning down the new hospital, the chief capitulated quite easily to pressure from Father Raynaud and the government. He officiated at the opening ceremony. I wasn't there. I heard about it in a letter from Anna. But that's part of a long story which you'll hear later. Suffice to say for the moment that the chief never had the new hospital burned down.

The Three Sons

HARRY ICEBOUND WAS A DOGRIB in his eighties who was having trouble urinating. The problem had developed slowly over a few years but had become much worse over several weeks. Examination revealed an enlarged prostate gland as the cause. I called in his wife who had been out in the waiting room. With Johnny interpreting, I did my best to explain his condition. After making a drawing of the gland and explaining how its enlargement caused obstruction of urinary flow, I explained that an operation was the only way to solve the problem. I also explained that if he didn't have an operation his kidneys could be destroyed by a gradual build-up of pressure. For the operation he would have to be flown to Edmonton a thousand miles to the south.

"Do you have any questions?" I asked through Johnny.

"No." Harry and his wife answered.

"Do you agree to having the operation?" I asked.

"Yes." Harry answered.

I called the hospital in Edmonton and arranged for Harry's admission for surgery in a week. Three hours later I received a radio call from one of the outlying settlements. A schoolteacher in the settlement was speaking for one of Harry Icebound's sons:

"Don't do anything until I get there."

During the day I received two similar messages from two more sons in two other settlements. Three days later there were three dog sleds leaning against Harry Icebound's shack, and thirty or so extra dogs chained outside the house. That morning Harry Icebound's three sons were waiting for me in the clinic when I arrived.

I brought the sons into my office and asked Johnny to translate. They had all travelled hundreds of miles by dogteam from their settlements over the last three days. They sat like captured wild creatures, with their heads cocked to the danger they felt all around them.

The one who appeared to be the eldest spoke. Johnny interpreted:

"We love the old man," he began. "Tell us about this operation," he continued.

Where the Balls Go

THE PHONE RANG at a little after midnight. It was Father Martine. His tone was panicky and his words were clipped with fear:

"We just brought in Rosie Bearskin on a stretcher by dogteam from Lynx River. She was bleeding all the way in!"

"Bleeding from where?" I asked.

Father Martine was an alarmist. I couldn't help being skeptical.

"From her vagina. She's been bleeding for six days."

It was probably simply a heavy period. But I knew it was pointless to even suggest that to Father Martine. For him everything was an emergency.

"O.K., I'll pick her up with the station wagon and bring her to the hospital. Where is she now?"

"At her mother's. Emilia Bearskin. House number 32."

"O.K.," I said. "I'll be there in a few minutes."

"Thank you, doctor. I'll come with her to the hospital."

Father Martine was the bush priest. He and Father Raynaud were the two tribal priests. I liked Father Martine. He really cared about the Dogribs. He lived alternately in the three outlying settlements; in each place he had a shack and a log chapel. Both priests had come to Canada twenty-five years ago as missionaries from a French order. They both spoke fluent Dogrib. Father Raynaud, the political priest, was gaunt and pale. Father Martine, the bush priest, was a huge, robust man with a booming voice.

Father Martine was an incorrigible hypochondriac. Not for himself. He never once asked me anything about his own health. He was only hypochondriacal about the health of the Dogribs. He would whip up their anxiety over the most insignificant symptoms. I was almost sure Rosie Bearskin's bleeding would be a case in point. But the problem is that you can never be sure. It could be a real vaginal hemorrhage. Knowing Father Martine it probably wasn't. But this was the way it always was when he was involved. From the moment he got word of anyone having a medical problem, he fanned their apprehension into florid panic. This sanguineous midnight dogsled trek was probably another example.

I dressed and headed out to the garage. It was fifty-five below zero. Coming out of the warm house, the cold air was shocking. The sky was crammed with stars. The dogs were howling more than usual. Maybe Father Martine was right. Maybe Rosie was dying. Or maybe someone else was. The northern lights flashed continuously across the sky, illuminating it like a cosmic pinball game with an Arctic theme. On the scoreboard nubile snowmaidens in skintight parkas leaned provocatively over neon igloos. It was one of the old games with no flippers. It was just you against fate. Just a question of how the balls bumped their way among the pins on their journey to the slot that sent them back under the board. Inevitably towards the end you might try to push the whole machine gently to keep the balls from the slot. Then TILT would flash on the board. All the lights would go dead. The remaining ball would plummet through the slot and thump below to where the balls rested between games. Finally the slot would close. For daring to shake the machine you lost all.

I prayed for TILT and cursed Father Martine in my Jewish heart. I prayed for a dybbuk to haunt his frozen chapels and frighten away his parishioners. I prayed for anything to avoid tearing myself out of bed at midnight like this.

I opened up the garage and started the station wagon. While the engine warmed up I went out to look at the driveway. It was a steep hill with the incline against you. As usual, tonight it was sheer ice. The garage was a converted tool shed. There was about a half an inch of space on each side of the station wagon as it went through the door. Nine months of the year the driveway was covered with ice. To get up the hill it usually took about a half an hour of coaxing the car with sand and iron grapplers underneath it, and neighbours pushing it from behind. At the same time as you pushed, you had to be wary of scratching the car against the door frame.

I had repeatedly asked headquarters in Yellowknife for a new garage, and for the incline of the driveway to be levelled. I reminded them that I was using the car for emergencies, and that having to take a half hour each time to get out of the garage was contrary to the public interest. The answer I received from Yellowknife was one that I was given for many similar and equally legitimate requests: "Dr. Griffin never complained about it," the Chief Maintenance Officer said.

Dr. Griffin was my immediate predecessor at Fort Collins. His name was always brought up at moments like these. His memory was held in reverence for his abject acceptance of all hardship. He was reputed to have been as acquiescent as I was perverse. Once when I phoned Yellowknife to complain that our cesspool was constantly backing up and filling our bathtub, I was told: "Dr. Griffin never complained about it."

Even the maintenance worker who eventually came out to fix the cesspool problem had a sanctimonious air. He was an old plumber of about seventy who told me about the first doctor who lived here: "At that time there was no road to Yellowknife. The doctor had to come into town by canoe in summer or by dog team in winter," the plumber said, covering his nose and mouth with one hand as he worked with the other. "Never mind shit in the bathtub," he continued, "that doctor had no bathtub at all."

"If you don't shut up you're going to get some shit in your face, you old geezer!" I said to myself. I was tired of being told I was a spoiled brat because I didn't want shit in my bathtub. This pompous plumber was intolerable, but I felt I had to stay beside him the whole time to make sure he did the work properly. Often the repair work done by maintenance men from Yellowknife was inadequate.

I sighed and threw some sand on the ice, and put some iron grapplers down on the tracks. I stepped on the gas. The sand raised a dust storm. The grapplers spun off and hit the walls of the garage. The station wagon stayed where it was. When he heard the wheels spinning, my nearest neighbour would usually come out and help. No sign of him tonight. I remembered he'd gone trapping in the bush and wouldn't be back for several weeks. The other neighbours only helped in the daytime. I looked around the garage for something else to put under the wheels besides the sand and grapplers. My glance fell on a pile of furniture. These were pieces of furniture that we had moved out of the house when we arrived because they were so depressing. I grabbed a headboard and placed it just in front of the back wheel. I got back in the car and stepped on the gas. I knew that this would be written up. Someday the government would send someone to take an inventory on the furniture in the doctor's house and he would find some of it in the garage. At the lynching, the frenzied crowd of bureaucrats would mutter indignantly: "Look what he does with the taxpayers' money! We buy him a bed, and what does he do? He sleeps on a mattress on the floor, and puts the headboard under his car wheels!"

That inevitable day of reckoning was far off. Now it was fifty-five below zero, and I had to pick up Rosie Bearskin. I had told them twenty times about the garage and incline. I pressed on the gas. The car rocked precariously over the headboard and shot up the hill. I drove to Rosie's mother's shack. Rosie looked fine. Better than Father Martine. He was getting older, and midnight dogsled trips were taking their toll.

I examined Rosie at the hospital. It was probably nothing more than a slightly prolonged period. She was forty-six years old. It was probably just the result of hormonal imbalance prior to menopause. It had been happening to her on and off for a year; it gave her menstrual periods of seven to eight days instead of four to five. This was the seventh day of one of those periods, and it was beginning to slow down. She had intended to see me about it the next time I came to Lynx River for a clinic. When Father Martine had asked about her health, she had mentioned the menstrual irregularity in a casual way. He had become very alarmed, and insisted she come immediately to Fort Collins to see me. Father Martine, while I examined Rosie, paced anxiously outside in the hall like an expectant father. He looked up apprehensively as I came out:

"So?" he queried dramatically.

"It's a slightly prolonged monthly period," I answered, "a little longer than usual." I continued, "It's probably because of hormonal imbalance that often occurs just before menopause. Her uterus is normal size. That makes anything else more serious very unlikely, but I will send her into Yellowknife over the next few days to see a gynecologist. They can do a dilatation and curettage just to make sure that nothing serious is being missed. We'll check her to make sure she's not anemic from these prolonged periods. What it will all probably come down to is the option of controlling these periods with hormones, or just waiting it out until menopause, as long as they don't get any worse. It's all something I could have arranged if I would have seen her next week at Lynx River, as she had planned before she spoke to you."

"Thank the Lord," Father Martine muttered fervently.

The pointed observation I had made about his unnecessary intervention hadn't penetrated. He was too entranced with the crisis he had created to hear it. He loved these medical dramas. It was so much more exciting for him than trying to wring emotion out of that tired old story that ended with the Crucifixion and Resurrection.

We brought Rosie back to her mother's shack. I drove Father Martine to Father Raynaud's where he stayed when he was in Fort Collins. Back home, I placed the headboard on the driveway, and eased the car into the garage. I put the headboard back among the furniture, carefully placing the tire marks facing inwards.

It was 2:23 a.m. The Arctic pinball game was quiet for the moment. All five of the heavy chrome balls had shouldered their way down the board with ever diminishing rebounds, shuddered impotently by the bottom pins, and thudded through the slot to the storage compartment below. As a child I'd always wondered what that compartment looked like.

I was wide awake but knew I had to get back to sleep to be able to face the morning clinic. I made some hot chocolate, and sat looking at the flag flapping and crackling in the wind outside the kitchen window.

The dogs were still howling more than usual. It wasn't for Rosie. Who was it for? Maybe I'd find out tomorrow. A welcome wave of fatigue suddenly overcame me. I headed for bed and for wherever the balls stayed between games.

As always, I went to sleep with a vague sense that the plug was still in the wall, just waiting for someone to put in a quarter and light up the board again. It could be at anytime. It might be a call from a nurse saying that someone was in labour or breathing quickly or slowly or not at all...

Lawrence Arrowmaker

LAWRENCE ARROWMAKER was two weeks old. I was examining him at Great Bear Creek in someone's shack. Great Bear Creek was one of the three outlying settlements where I did monthly visits. I hadn't delivered him because his birth had required a caesarean section which had been done in Yellowknife, so this was the first time I was seeing him. I knew his mother Louise well. She was the lay dispenser in the settlement. The lay dispenser in each settlement is given a manual on emergency medical care, a bag of medical supplies and drugs, and a radio set to call the nearest doctor. The government pays them a salary and sends them for a preliminary training course in a medical centre for several weeks. In Louise's case the radio was kept in the schoolteacher's shack because Louise spoke very little English. During clinics in the settlements the lay dispensers would act as assistants, and I would try as much as possible to teach them while we worked. I enjoyed working with Louise. She was bright and conscientious, and the people in the settlement respected and trusted her.

Louise was proud of Lawrence. He was her first child. The delivery had been difficult. But that was passed. Now she could enjoy taking care of him. She undressed him for what we both thought would be a routine exam. At one glance it was evident something was seriously wrong with Lawrence. He was breathing much too fast. I listened with my stethoscope. The breath sounds were much too faint on the left side of the chest. The heart sounds were shifted to the right. Something was causing his left lung to collapse.

I took Lawrence back with me to Fort Collins. There was no room for Louise in the plane because I had to bring in another patient with heart failure. Luckily Louise wasn't breastfeeding, and Lawrence could be fed by bottle. I had the plane wait at Fort Collins while I did a chest X-ray. It showed a shift of the heart toward the right. It confirmed that there was something in the left side of the chest other than the lungs and the heart. Something was obstructing the function of the left lung and causing Lawrence to struggle for breath. I brought the baby back into the plane and flew on with him to Yellowknife.

In Yellowknife, an X-ray taken after we gave the baby some contrast material to drink in his milk, showed that his stomach was up in the left side of his chest. The baby had been born with a defect in the diaphragm which had allowed the stomach to shift up into the lung area. As a result the left lung was partially collapsed, and the lungs, heart and trachea were pushed over to the right. If this went on uncorrected, the function of the right lung would be gradually impeded as well—and Lawrence would die. A defect in the diaphragm is a fairly common congenital condition and can be corrected surgically. This was one of those happy instances where medical technology could provide an instant cure. The stomach is returned to its anatomical bed and the defect in the diaphragm is repaired. Lawrence Arrowmaker, an infant who would have died of internal suffocation, would be saved.

Lawrence had to be flown a thousand miles south to Edmonton for the surgery. Ordinarily a nurse would have accompanied him. In this instance I chose to go with him. For some time I had wanted to go down to Edmonton and meet the doctors at the hospital to whom I was sending patients. The government had agreed in principle to this idea and was willing to pay for my trip and arrange for doctors from Yellowknife to cover Fort Collins for emergencies. I thought this was a perfect time to carry out the plan. I would bring Lawrence Arrowmaker down to Edmonton and visit the hospital at the same time.

I flew down to Edmonton with Lawrence in my arms. We were picked up at the airport by an ambulance. I brought Lawrence up to the pediatric ward of the hospital and discussed his case with his doctors. The operation was scheduled for eleven the next morning. I made arrangements to tour the hospital until noon when the operation would be over.

I checked into a hotel. I felt elated. I was saving this baby's life. He was now safely in the hospital. And I was safely in a city where I had no medical responsibilities and could live for a night like an ordinary person. It felt strange. Sitting in this hotel room, it was hard for me to believe that we lived in a little house surrounded by howling dogs and a perpetually moaning wind. After six months of being on constant call, I savoured having this night off.

As I was scanning the movie page in the newspaper, my room telephone rang. I couldn't believe it. It was a nurse from Snowdrift on the line. Snowdrift was a settlement in another area that I covered when their doctor was away. I had been traced a thousand miles to answer this emergency call. It should have been answered by the doctors in Yellowknife who were replacing me. The nurse was asking for authorization to order a plane to send a patient with appendicitis to Yellowknife. Someone in Fort Collins had given her the number of the hospital in Edmonton where Lawrence was, and said I could be reached there. The hospital in Edmonton had given her the number of the hotel. After all the nurse's effort to reach me, I didn't have the heart to tell her to call the doctors in Yellowknife and authorize the flight to Snowdrift. I called the airline in Yellowknife and authorized the flight. I called the hospital in Yellowknife and advised the doctor on call the patient would be coming. I called back the nurse in Snowdrift to tell her everything was arranged. All these calls took an hour. It was now too late to go to a movie.

I tried to go for a walk along the main street of the city, but suddenly felt exhausted. The strain of that last hour of phone calls about the patient from Snowdrift was more than I could take on a day which had started with a flight to Great Bear Creek for a clinic at six in the morning. I returned to my hotel room feeling very lonely, and wishing I was with my family in the little house among the howling dogs and the moaning wind.

In the morning I was given a tour of the hospital and met the doctors to whom I had been referring patients for six months. I visited some patients from Fort Collins who were in the hospital and were very surprised to see me. In Fort Collins I was an outsider. Here they greeted me as a relic from home. At noon I went to the surgical recovery room to check on Lawrence Arrowmaker.

Lawrence was dead.

During the operation on the diaphragm, the heart is pushed aside for the surgeon to have room to work. Manipulating the heart in this way can cause disturbances in cardiac rhythm which are usually easily controlled. During the operation the cardiac monitor had become detached. The heart at one point is completely covered with drapes. During that time Lawrence had a cardiac arrest which went unobserved because of the detached electrode. By the time it was noticed, Lawrence had irreparable brain damage. There was no response to repeated attempts at resuscitation.

Allowing the monitor to become detached was gross negligence. The doctors and the hospital should be sued, but this seemed of little consequence for the moment. That would come later. What I had to face now was telling Louise Arrowmaker that Lawrence was dead. Nobody here understood that I had taken this little baby from his mother and told her that I would bring him home well. I was bringing him home dead.

I phoned Yellowknife and asked the operator to hook me up to the radio in Great Bear Creek. As the operator made the connection, I could see the settlement appearing below me as it does when I approach it by plane: a tiny clump of shacks and tents huddled on a vast expanse of snow. I knew the radio was in the schoolteacher's cabin. As usual it was taking the operator a long time to make the connection. Usually the wait annoyed me. This time I was grateful for it.

The schoolteacher in whose cabin the radio was kept was a young man named John Griffin. He was one of those people who is born mature. John was twenty-three years old, but handled himself with the insight and clarity that might have come to an astute person after another twenty or thirty years. He was the only white person in the settlement. Three years ago he had been sent by the government to teach school, and had arrived to find there was no schoolhouse and nowhere for him to live. With the Dogribs' help he built a schoolhouse and a cabin to live in. He spoke fluent Dogrib. The people liked him and trusted him. They would often ask his advice. I was grateful that he would be the translator.

The telephone connection was made. John was in the schoolhouse. Someone was going to get him. They knew the call was from Edmonton and that it was from the doctor. They knew it must be about Louise's baby. Everybody knew everything about everybody in Great Bear Creek. They had probably gone for Louise at the same time. As I waited for John to take the phone, I wished I were a schoolteacher like him and didn't have to live all the time with life and death consequences. As I waited for him to come to the phone, I wished I had never become a doctor.

Misdemeanors

IT'S ELEVEN O'CLOCK Saturday morning and it's still pitch black outside. It's forty below zero. The Canadian flag in front of the town hall is flapping madly in the wind. It has been an exhausting week. I'm hoping it will continue to be a peaceful day at home in the dark with my family. The phone rings: "Hello," I answer. I'm hoping it's for Lenore. It almost never is.

"Hello, Doctor. This is Frank Washee speaking. There's a man with frostbite in his foot stranded in a hunting camp about a hundred and forty miles from here. We left him with someone to keep a fire and feed him, and came in by dogteam to get help. Can you get a plane to evacuate him?"

"Yes, I can," I answer. "I'll meet you at the hospital and you can show me where it is on the map."

I meet Frank at the hospital and he shows me the location of the camp on an area map on the wall of my office. I call the charter airplane company that serves the hospital. They tell me that since the men are not at a fixed settlement, I need to ask the police to send out a search plane. I call the police, and they say that if the Indians know where the camp is—it's not a search—and that I should call a charter company.

Under police duress, and with the assurance that the Dogribs can find the hunting camp from the air, the charter company agrees to send a plane. Because it involves a stretcher, they are sending a Twin Otter, which is a larger plane than the usual single engine planes we usually use. An hour later a plane arrives in front of my house. The flight has attracted the whole village to my doorstep. This time no one has packages for me to deliver, because I have a destination where nobody lives. Nonetheless, it's a festive atmosphere. It's a big plane and everyone's excited. I get in with my medical bag and a stretcher. Johnny, my interpreter, comes with me, and an old Dogrib of about eighty, who Johnny says can find the camp.

A Twin Otter has two engines with two propellers. It takes a co-pilot to operate it. We get in behind the two pilots. A sign flashes over their heads. NO SMOKING. FASTEN YOUR SEAT BELTS.

We have no seat belts because we have no seats. We are sitting on the floor as the seats have been removed to accommodate a stretcher. The old Dogrib takes a long inhalation on his pipe. The two pilots have a solemn contempt for everything that is happening. For them native people are a drunken sub-race. A doctor who would live among them is either not a real doctor, or one that was probably disbarred, or some kind of derelict. They stare ahead sullenly. They are confident that the old man will never find one tent down there somewhere in hundreds of miles of featureless bush.

We fly for about forty minutes in what we know is the general direction of the camp. The old man takes his pipe out of his mouth and speaks quietly to Johnny in Dogrib.

"Turn right," Johnny tells the pilot.

Ten minutes later the old man puts down his pipe and speaks again to Johnny.

"Turn left," Johnny tells the pilot.

There is nothing below us but endless sheets of stunted fir trees and lakes. About five minutes later we see a wisp of smoke among the trees. About thirty seconds later we see the smoke is coming from a flap in the roof of a grey canvas tent. On the snow beside the tent are two dozen dark spots that stir as we circle, and stand up and bark defiantly as we close in for a landing.

The frostbite has not yet become gangrenous. The only problems are his dogteam and sled and the caribou he has shot. He wants me to take them with us on the plane. It's a big plane. There's enough space. The problem is that it's against regulations to transport public property on a government flight. I think about it, but not for long. I turn to Johnny and say:

"Let's get the dogs and sled and caribou on."

Six months later I got a call from a government official from headquarters in Yellowknife asking me the names of all persons having anything to do with the flight. He didn't ask me about the dogs and sleds and caribou. They were building up the case with testimony from anyone who had been on the plane: the pilots, Johnny, the old man, and the frostbitten hunter. Johnny would be afraid to lie. He would lose his job. I couldn't blame him. He would be right in assuming that the pilots would have told the truth. It would all come out when they closed in. It was only one of my many misdemeanours. I was constantly guilty of breaking regulations. It began the first week when I had given Richard Zoe, the man who had been cursed by the black magician, a ride home from Yellowknife the night an Arctic owl had broken his windshield. I never realized till the end how much I was hated by the people at headquarters in Yellowknife. Headquarters was run by an immigrant doctor who was working in the north because his licence wasn't recognized anywhere else. His name was Dr. Ben Youssef. If he hated anything more than he hated me, it was the north and the native people. He had once said to me in an argument:

"Why do you care so much for a band of savages?"

His hatred dated from his first sight of me. My casual dress and longish hair were an insult to his conception of a doctor. For him the suspicion my appearance engendered was confirmed quite early. In his terms I proved to be a troublemaker. On my first day in Fort Collins I discovered that bacteriological specimens were being sent to a lab in Edmonton one thousand miles south. The results would arrive two weeks later. This was useless for any decision in treatment. It would only tell you when it was too late whether what you did was right or not. Immediately I began to do something more rational. I sent the bacterial cultures to the local hospital in Yellowknife and got answers in one or two days. On my ninth day of the job I received a phone call from Dr. Youssef:

"I have a bill here for bacteriological cultures from the hospital in Yellowknife," he said accusingly.

"That's because I sent cultures there," I answered and added, "and got very good and very prompt service."

"We send cultures to the provincial lab in Edmonton. They are done at no cost to us."

"That may be so. But it's a useless service for us. They're a thousand miles away. We get the results two weeks later——"

"That didn't impede your predecessors from administering quality care——"

"Whatever kind of care they were giving, it was without the help of bacterial cultures. A result received two weeks after——"

"Doctor, any bills for bacteriological cultures that I receive from

Yellowknife subsequent to this conversation will be deducted from your salary—"

The phone clicked closed on his side.

There were about twenty employees in the regional headquarters in Yellowknife. They sat in an office dreaming of re-appointment in southern Canada. Often one of them would phone the hospital at eight-thirty in the morning to see if I were in the clinic working. If I wasn't there, they would mark it down and store that information away for my ultimate bureaucratic lynching. Between eight and nine in the morning I was often doing house calls on old bedridden patients. That was irrelevant. What was important was that I wasn't there.

My second early battle with Dr. Ben Youssef was over public health visits. According to my job description, in addition to being the medical officer for Fort Colins, I was also the health inspector for a town called Providence which was about a hundred and fifty miles away.

I was supposed to visit Providence every two months for public health inspection. It was a little town of about seven hundred people. I was supposed to check if the toilets in the school and the town's one restaurant were clean, and certify that the restaurant's kitchen was clean. I was also supposed to take a water sample from the town's reservoir. The nurses in the nursing station took samples monthly. The samples I was taking were no different from those the nurses took.

This bi-monthly health inspection had been planned by a bureaucratic madman sitting at a desk somewhere in southern Canada, who had no comprehension of the public health and medical needs of communities in the Northwest Territories. To perform this insane trip six times a year, the doctor at Fort Collins has to leave hospitalized patients and cancel the daily clinic. During the day he is unable to make emergency flights to the outlying settlements should the need arise.

It was also decreed that the doctor must travel by car for this trip. For any other similar trip of a hundred and fifty miles the doctor could charter a plane. The mad bureaucrat in the south had decided this trip should be made by car. It meant leaving early in the morning and coming home late in the evening —to check the kitchen and toilets of one restaurant and the toilets in the school six times a year. It was the

kind of inspection that might occur in a school or restaurant in southern Canada once in many years, if at all.

Of course the restaurant owners and the school principal hated
the doctor. Six times a year he would appear and have to be shown
the same tired toilets and refrigerators by the same tired people. With
the scarcity of medical care in the north, these people could reason-
ably question a doctor being paid to examine their toilets six times a
year.

I went on that trip twice in nine months. On the second trip I
noticed some slightly tainted meat in the bottom of one of the refrigerators in the restaurant. It had fallen in between two meat racks and
probably gone unnoticed. I brought it to the owner's attention, being
careful to tell him that it wasn't at all serious, and that I didn't intend
to report it.

I never did write down anything about the meat. The restaurant
owner did, however, write a long letter to Dr. Ben Youssef reporting
that I had brought my family on the trip. This was true. I had felt that
if I was going to be torn away from Fort Collins for a day on this
useless quest, I might as well take my family for a drive. This was
against regulations. The restaurant owner's letter was added to the
file Dr. Ben Youssef kept on me. In the civil service when people want
to get rid of you they keep a file on you and record all misdemeanours.
The process is called "writing-up" someone. Because of the opposition I had been voicing about moving the hospital to the new town,
Dr. Ben Youssef was writing me up with a passion that produces giant
novels.

A few days after my second and last public health visit to Providence, a health inspector knocked on our house door and asked my
wife, Lenore, if he could inspect our house. This in itself was as-
tounding. Why couldn't this health inspector visit Providence as well
as Fort Collins? After he left, Lenore called me at the hospital. She
was alarmed:

"The health inspector said there was some poisonous hydrogen
sulphide gas seeping up from our basement! He said it could be fatal!
He said we should call Yellowknife and have them fix it immediately!"

I called Yellowknife and spoke to the director of maintenance for
government housing. The answer I received was the same one I always

received when I called to report any maintenance problem: "Dr. Griffin never complained about that," responded the director of maintenance.

"Dr. Griffin has nothing to do with it," I countered. "I don't even have anything to do with it. He's your health inspector. And he says it's poisonous gas that can kill us!"

"Dr. Griffin was there three years and he never said a word about it," the director answered.

Scars

ZENO WAS A FREE TRADER. The term was applied to someone on a native reservation who owned a store that was independent of the Hudson's Bay Company. In colonial times the King of England had made the Hudson's Bay Company the rulers of the Northwest Territories. The company was no longer the government, but it still controlled the economic life of most of the Dogribs. Those who lived by trapping kept a running bill—at compound interest—with the Bay store for food and supplies until the trapping season. After the trapping season they would come back from the bush and sell the company their furs against what they owed in their account. The company shipped the furs to southern Canada to the fur auctions, where they were sold for many times the amount they had paid the native trappers.

Zeno's was a true general store: he stocked just about everything, and anything he didn't have he could get for the right price within reasonable time. Attached to the store, and also owned by Zeno, were the only restaurant and the only poolhall in town. Come to think of it, Zeno ran the only shopping mall in the stunted tree zone.

Since drinking was officially prohibited in Fort Collins by the Council of Elders of the tribe, there was no bar in the settlement. Zeno's poolhall and restaurant was the only hangout. It was like the saloon in a cowboy movie. In the fifty-below zero world of Fort Collins, Zeno's restaurant and poolhall, with its twenty-year-old Wurlitzer with hit parade selections of three years ago, was the only place to connect with the outside world— not the official outside world as it was reached through the church, the tribal council and the government, but the unofficial world that Dogribs had seen everyday and come back to tell about.

Zeno, with his tainted hot dogs and hamburgers in stale buns, was trading in whiffs of non-reservation living. Consequently he and his store were shunned by most of the white people living in Fort Collins. For most of the schoolteachers, police, maintenance workers and nuns it was as if Zeno's didn't exist. The Hudson's Bay store with its traditional role in the colonial hierarchy was a more comfortable place for white people to buy a pair of gloves or socks. They went to the Bay store even though Zeno often had the same articles at a cheaper price. Zeno's smelled of the outside world and all its options. It was too threatening a place for people who profited by the status quo in Fort Collins.

Zeno was a Greek whose restaurant in a Greek town had been swallowed up, along with half the town, by an earthquake. He had made his way with his family to Edmonton, and worked in other Greeks' restaurants until he had saved enough money to head up north, and set up the only restaurant in Fort Collins. From it had sprung the only poolhall and the only free-trading store. In Fort Collins Zeno was clearly an outsider. He functioned from outside and between the lines. As a result he had an outsider's clarity of vision. To that insight was coupled his own particular streetfighter's acumen. When Zeno talked to me about Fort Collins I always listened intently. Here he was talking about Father Raynaud: "Raynaud's going to get you," Zeno said shaking his forefinger at me emphatically. "I've seen doctors come and go. When he doesn't like a doctor—" he paused and then whispered, "they don't last very long!" His forefinger and thumb went from pointing to me to twirling his mustache, and then became part of a fist that pounded gently but emphatically on the store counter in front of him. "He's furious about your trying to block moving the hospital to the new town," Zeno continued. "He knows you spoke to the chief about organizing opposition."

"So what if he knows—"

"So what?" Zeno asked incredulously, "I can't believe you're that naive! He wants the new town, right?"

"Right."

"And you're against the new town, right?"

"Right."

"So it's simple. He's going to turn all the people of the town against you—and get you out of here. He's already started. He's being making points against you on the death of that kid in Edmonton. You left with the kid, and the kid came back dead. Then there's those two old guys who died in the first few weeks you came—Michel Trapper and Samuel Erasmus."

"They were ninety-five percent dead the first day I got here. They—"

"You don't have to waste your time telling me about it. Of course I know that. But that's only two of us. And I'm a 'non-person' here; despised for making an honest living. That leaves you. And how long have you been here? A year? And how long has Raynaud been here? Twenty-five years. And he speaks to them in Dogrib with all the sneaky power that someone's own language can have on them. And he has the fear of hell on his side. You can strut around with your stethoscope, and order airplanes every ten minutes, but all you can do about a trip to hell is delay it. They believe that in the end whether they go there or not depends upon the balance in their account with Raynaud."

Walking home from Zeno's I thought about the two old men who had died. They were both permanent residents of the hospital. Michel Trapper was so old the features of his face were barely discernable in the maze of his wrinkles. With the Dogrib nursing assistants translating, I used to talk with him when I was making rounds in the hospital. Particularly on Sundays when there was no clinic, and rounds in the hospital were very relaxed, I had listened to stories he told of the old ways of living and hunting. He had a tumour of the bladder, which had been operated on several times, and he had been left with a permanent urinary catheter. His wife had died many years ago. His children lived in distant settlements, and would visit him at Christmas and Easter when the whole tribe gathered in Fort Collins. He died one night in his sleep. Probably a heart attack. In other words he just died. His time ran out.

The second man, Samuel Erasmus, had an inoperable cancer of the lung which spread to his liver and brain. It would have been cruel as well as futile to send him to the hospital in Yellowknife. He passed those last few days among his family and the people he knew, instead of in some strange and terrifying place. The night he died was my first exposure to the Dogrib way of dealing with death. Even though he was comatose and didn't hear a thing they were saying, his family and friends came to his bedside, and placing their hands on his in turn, rendered long wailing accounts of Samuel's virtues as a husband, father and tribal member. They told tales of his prowess as a hunter. They told stories of his knowledge of the wilderness, and his strength and courage in dealing with it at all times. The moment he died they began the arduous task of digging a grave in the frozen ground. It took a dozen men a whole day of digging in the permafrost, in forty below zero cold, to dig a hole deep enough to place a coffin in.

Father Raynaud was telling the people I should have sent him to Yellowknife. He knows better than that. But as Zeno says the truth is not the issue here. For Raynaud I'm in the way. For him my being in the way was wrong, and getting me out of the way is right. That bastard! Blaming me for the deaths of those old men! And for Lawrence Arrowmaker's death!

I felt really low. But not as low as the day I sent my own four month old son Allen out with severe dehydration from a gastroenteritis that was near fatal. I sent Allen out to the University Hospital in Edmonton a thousand miles south of us. A nurse went with him to regulate the intravenous fluid he was receiving in flight, and my wife Lenore went as the one parent escort the government regulations allow for. To this day Lenore gets angry, and can't really look at me, when she remembers how I sent them out alone, and didn't go with them. She's absolutely right. Of course I should have gone with them. I was stupid. I made the decision thinking as the doctor at Fort Collins, and not as a father and husband. My reasoning at the time was based on the fact that the government payed for one parent to go with a child as an escort. I could pay for myself, but I felt that as the doctor in the settlement, I would never again be able to face parents in the same situation who couldn't afford to do what I could. Also, I was new on the job, and felt guilty about leaving my post, since I was going to be superfluous in Allen's medical care. In retrospect I could have asked for coverage of Fort Collins from doctors in Yellowknife, as I learned was possible several months later, when I took Lawrence

Arrowmaker, the baby who died in surgery, down to Edmonton. Beyond all these theoretical considerations, the net result was that for very superficial reasons, I sent Lenore with Allen a thousand miles away, to fight for his life in an unknown hospital in a strange city. Every time I think of it I cringe at my stupidity and callousness. On top of everything else, I had made a mistake in Allen's treatment which was a major factor in the severity of his dehydration. At one point he had seemed to be getting slightly better. At that point one of the older nurses suggested giving him a clear soup. I knew it was a sentimental and scientifically unsound idea. But I wanted to believe he was better. An hour after eating the soup he began to vomit and have diarrhea again. A doctor at Edmonton told Lenore that the soup had played a role in his subsequent deterioration. Lenore could barely speak about it on the phone. It was too horrible to convey.

Walking home from Zeno's, I was thinking of that morning when Allen was being evacuated with Lenore to Edmonton, and I could hear the plane approaching. I ran to the chief maintenance man's house to find out where a runway had been cleared. The site of the runway would sometimes change because of snowdrifts and wind conditions. The chief maintenance man was a white man who was an appointee of the town manager. I had never had any previous dealings with him, but since the town manager and Father Raynaud saw me as a trouble-maker, I knew the chief maintenance man would feel the same way.

I could hear the plane approaching. In my haste to find out where the runway was, I stepped into the chief maintenance man's house without taking off my snowboots. He made a big fuss about it: "Didn't you ever learn to take off your snowboots before you come into someone's house?" he snarled derisively.

"You're right. I'm sorry," I answered hastily. "But my kid is critically ill. He's being evacuated. Time's very important here. It's a matter of life and death. I just want to know where the runway's been cleared—"

"But you could have stood outside until I came to the door," the chief maintenance man persisted. The plane engine was sounding louder and closer, and I still didn't know where the runway was. The chief maintenance man continued relentlessly: "You didn't have to come in here with your boots all covered with snow and drip it all over the place!"

I grabbed a broom which was near the door and swept away the small amount of snow my boots had carried in. "O.K.? Is that all right now you son of a bitch?!" I yelled. "Now where is the goddamn runway?" I grabbed him by the collar. "If you don't tell me in the next two seconds I'm going to kill you!"

I was well written up for that episode by the chief maintenance man—with Dr. Ben Youssef's help. I was described as displaying behaviour not befitting a medical officer. The fact that Allen was critically ill and the maintenance man was withholding vital information was never considered relevant.

During the time Allen and Lenore were down in the hospital in Edmonton, while I was working I had no one to take care of my four year old son Mark. Because there was no one I could leave him with, I had to take him with me on a medical trip to a settlement. I was written up for taking him on that flight: I was criticized for having a member of my family accompanying me while on medical duty, and using public transport for family members.

I was being written up passionately, voluminously and endlessly for what was essentially a civilian court martial, which would occur when renewal of my contract came up after a year on the job. I was starting to feel weary of constantly being on trial, with no one to speak in my defence except me. It added to the strain of being the only doctor—and a relatively inexperienced one at that. At times I would feel bad about my inexperience. My mistake with Allen was an example. But I also knew there was no one with more experience who had wanted to come here, and I was doing the best I could. But walking home from Zeno's that night, after hearing that Father Raynaud was blaming me for deaths for which I was innocent, I was tempted to knock on Raynaud's door and cause one for which I would be guilty.

Walking home in the cold with the dogs howling, I thought of Lenore sitting beside Allen in the hospital in Edmonton, and Allen getting intravenous fluid through a vein in his head. She had sat there knowing I was partly to blame for his condition. And I had let them go down there alone.

Lenore had tolerated the isolation and hardship of living in Fort Collins so that I could do the kind of medicine I wanted to do. But sitting there in Edmonton alone with Allen critically ill was beyond tolerance. Allen recovered uneventfully over the next few days. Thank God.

Wounds in the body heal by scarring. Marriages have theirs scars as well. Over the years scars can fade and become less noticeable. But they are scars nonetheless, and the pain they commemorate is nonetheless pain.

The Meeting

THE CONTROVERSY over the new hospital in the new town had escalated. Father Raynaud and the town manager were for it. Dr. Ben Youssef, my boss in Yellowknife, was for it. The white maintenance workers and most of the schoolteachers were for it. Only the Dogribs were against it.

The new town was ten miles from the lake. The government built houses on the site and offered them to the Dogribs at a nominal rent. The houses were bright and new, and had indoor toilets and oil heating. There were no takers. The government responded by moving the school to the new town. They figured that would begin the migration. No one moved. The children had to be bussed to the new school in the empty village. The government lodged the white schoolteachers in this first batch of unclaimed houses.

Construction began on the hospital. Father Raynaud, the town manager, Dr. Ben Youssef and the government reasoned that the old people, who were dependent on the hospital, would want to move to the new town once the hospital was there. They reasoned further that respect for the elders would then trigger a mass move. The authorities had miscalculated. The old people were the strongest objectors. Nobody moved.

For the government there was no turning back. The contracts had gone out. Materials had been ordered. The digging had begun. Father Raynaud, the town manager and Dr. Ben Youssef arranged a meeting between the government and the Dogribs. They invited the deputy director of Northern Health and Welfare.

The Department of Northern Health and Welfare vehicles are

bright red, with gold government insignia painted on the two front doors. A fleet of these cars arrived the day of the meeting. There was even a red limousine for the deputy director—who couldn't make it and had sent an assistant deputy director in his place. The meeting was held in the town hall. There was a heavy snow falling, so the government maintenance men decided to put the limousine in a garage during the meeting. The garage nearest the town hall was mine. After much skidding down the incline of the driveway, the limousine was parked in my garage.

The meeting began with a speech by the assistant deputy director of Northern Health and Welfare, who spoke through an interpreter. He began by apologizing for the deputy director's absence, explaining that he was unavoidably detained. He spoke about the great strides that had been achieved in native health since the present government took power, and then introduced Dr. Ben Youssef.

Dr. Ben Youssef had the lights in the hall turned off, and began to show some overhead projections of the building plans of the new hospital. He had barely started when someone opened the lights. Chief Drybones rose from the crowd and interrupted him. Ignoring Dr. Ben Youssef he turned toward the assistant deputy director, speaking through an interpreter:

"I am the chief of the Dogrib nation." he said and paused for effect: "I regret that your chief did not come. I would have explained to him that the purpose of this meeting was not to show drawings of a hospital the Dogribs do not want. It was to hear our objections to this plan, and then give us the assurance that it would not be carried out. After all, if the hospital is for us, and we don't want it, why would your chief persist in building it for us? Moving our village will destroy our way of living. Moving the hospital to a place where no one wants to live is even a more serious error than moving the school. In emergencies lives will be lost."

The chief sat down and the assistant deputy rose and answered through an interpreter: "I'm afraid you've been misinformed. To my knowledge this was not to be a meeting to discuss the pros and cons of moving your village. That decision was made a long time ago. It was a decision that bears no debate. It's a move dictated by public health. Your village is built on rock. It makes it impossible to build a real sewage system. You can't lay down pipes in rock—"

"Yellowknife was built on rock," the chief interjected.

It was true. The white mining town of Yellowknife a hundred miles down the lake had been built on the same rock.

"I know for a fact they have indoor toilets in Yellowknife," the chief continued. "You may have used one in your stop there. If you didn't, you should have. You would have made a better speech."

While the crowd laughed at this last remark, the chief paused for effect. Looking first at the audience, and then at the assistant deputy, he said slowly and firmly: "We will burn down your hospital."

After the meeting, while trying to get out of my garage, the driver scraped both front doors of the limousine. They were both long, deep scrapes that rendered the golden Northern Health and Welfare insignia on both doors into unintelligible abstractions. The driver himself was one of the maintenance officials with whom I'd argued about the garage and driveway for an entire year. A group of Dogribs with large smiles on their faces pushed the mangled car up the incline. Lenore, watching with the kids from our living room window, had the biggest smile of all.

Sarah One-Foot-in-Hell

IT'S SUNSET and I'm looking out on Great Slave Lake from our back window, I'm watching some kids skating on a little creek that feeds into the lake. We're leaving Fort Collins tomorrow. I'm writing some notes about our final day here. My mind keeps wandering back to the first day we arrived. We had only been here five minutes, when two police officers had knocked on the door. They were carrying some bones in a plastic bag:

"Are these human?" they had asked.

I examined the bones. They weren't human. They were probably bones from something like a bobcat or a young caribou.

"I'm not sure what they are," I said, "but I know they're not human."

"We have to find some human bones fast," one officer said.

"Why?" I asked.

"About two days ago a bear dug up a fresh grave and went off with the body. It was a lady named Sarah One-Foot-in-Hell who died a week ago. The whole village is in a state of panic. They believe that until her body is found, her spirit will roam around and cause trouble. The chief asks us about five times a day if we found it yet."

Over the next week the police kept coming with bags of bones. None of them were human. On the tenth day a trapper found some well licked human bones that certainly looked like they could have belonged to a frail old lady. I was happy to say the search was over. Sarah One-Foot-in-Hell was reburied and a great party and drum dance were held in the Community Centre to celebrate the event. At the party I learned that the family name was originally Two-Feet-in-Hell, but her husband had found his name too sombre and changed it. One-Foot-in-Hell still linked them to the family, but left a bit more grounds for optimism.

We were leaving because my contract wasn't being renewed. In a government job like mine not being rehired was equal to being fired. I could have protested, but I didn't care any longer. The new hospital was almost finished. Many Dogribs had begun to move into the new town. The chief had made a great protest speech at that meeting about the hospital, but neither he nor anyone else ever burned it down. I was told later in a letter from Anna that the chief laid the cornerstone in the opening ceremony.

Dr. Ben Youssef had blocked my being rehired by stating that I had demonstrated medical incompetence in trying to obstruct the hospital move. His position was that in trying to block a plan that was conducive to improved health of the tribe, I was counter-productive as a medical officer, and thus incompetent. He also appended a long list of the people other than patients to whom I had extended public transport, and ended with a graphic description of the headboard with the tiremarks on it.

I didn't protest because I was exhausted. I didn't want the contract renewed. I didn't want to live in the new town. I would miss Anna. I would miss Johnny. I would miss the cold night sky crammed with stars. I would even miss the howling of the dogs and the moaning of the wind. But I wouldn't miss Father Raynaud, the town manager, Dr. Ben Youssef or the chief. I didn't want to live in their new suburb. Nor did I want my children to grow up in it.

San Pedro

Franklin

MY PLANE LANDED in El Paso a few minutes after midnight. I was picked up at the airport by the director of the hospital and an Apache driver. I couldn't make out any details in the darkness, but had a sense of a gradual climb from flatlands to hills to mountains.

"The chief uses the hospital as his personal whipping boy," the director was saying. "It's his scapegoat to vent resentment against white people in general," he continued. "It's a shame because the hospital is one institution that is really there for their own good."

Four previous directors had been fired in less than three years. Several doctors had been fired as well. I could tell he was going to be fired next. And soon. He was completely out of control. He spoke as if the Apache driver didn't exist at all. His anxiety didn't move me. My fingers had been burnt in Fort Collins. I would stay out of politics. This had all been going on before I got here, and would be going on after I left. As he droned on, I tried to catch a glimpse of what was speeding by in the night.

When I had seen the end coming in Fort Collins, I had phoned down to the Indian Health Service in United States and asked for a job in the American southwest. I was offered a post in San Pedro, an Apache reservation in New Mexico. It was a two-doctor hospital. After a year alone in Fort Collins it sounded luxurious to have another doctor to work with. The day before I arrived, the other doctor left for an operation on his knee and didn't return for three months. Two days after I arrived, a week long annual festival began, during which thousands of Indians from all over the southwest poured into the village. The population swelled from two thousand to twelve thousand. The festival celebrated an annual female puberty rite. Male dancers in black body paint and elaborate headdresses, danced all night around mammoth bonfires fifty feet in height. The girls danced all night in front of a ceremonial tent. Periodically they would stop and confer good luck on people by touching them on the forehead with bee pollen. It all might have wrought good luck for everyone else, but for me the week was a sleepless kaleidoscopic blur which included two births and three deaths among the visitors. The deaths were all consequences of drinking: a car accident while driving drunk, a stabbing in a drunken brawl, and an alcoholic who bled to death from ruptured esophageal veins.

As we pulled into the hospital, I noticed a huge H painted on the parking lot just beside the entrance to the Emergency. I wondered what it stood for. The director had talked himself into an uneasy sleep. From the way he was mumbling and moaning, I could tell he was dreaming about the chief. I thought of asking the driver, but decided I would find out in time.

I found out what the H stood for sooner than I'd thought I would. We arrived at San Pedro about two in the morning, and I was given a key to the departed doctor's house. I fell asleep immediately and was wakened at seven in the morning by a phone call from the hospital. Someone was asking me to come immediately to the emergency room. A man who had been changing a giant tractor tire in the tribal garage had been pinned to the ceiling by the tire when it had blown off the changing apparatus. It had carried him fifteen feet up in the air and crushed him against the ceiling. He had fallen to the cement floor of the garage and the heavy tire landed on him and crushed him a second time. He was comatose and in profound shock, with a barely discernible blood pressure, and a rapid and faint pulse. He was bleeding internally. I poured intravenous fluid into him and called for blood for transfusion. He was rapidly bleeding to death. His only hope would be instant diagnosis of the source of the bleeding—with immediate repair of the arteries involved. Suddenly his blood pressure dropped beyond measure, his pulse disappeared and his heart stopped. It was then that I learned what the H stood for. An airforce helicopter was landing on it. A team in battle fatigues leaped out of the helicopter. They had been called at the same time as me, because the nurses had known the patient would need evacuation. The help was elegant. There was a doctor and three medic assistants. The equipment was superb. We worked for an hour trying to get the patient's heart to beat but didn't succeed. When I declared him dead, and rolled the cardiac defibrillator aside, a wail rose from everywhere at once: relatives of the dead man came wailing in from the waiting room; Apache nurses and nursing attendants and cleaners were wailing. My first case in San Pedro. I tried to speak to his wife. Understandably, she wasn't interested in anything I had to say. Her husband, who had left for work this morning alive and well was now dead. Nothing I could say was of interest to her—neither my explanations nor my condolences.

I stepped outside and watched the helicopter take off. It was from an American airforce base whose hospital served as our back-up for surgery and intensive care. The base was at Almagordo, at the edge of the White Sands Desert, where the atomic bomb had been tested prior to its use on Hiroshima.

I had come down to San Pedro to see what it was like. If I felt it was a good place for us to live, the family would follow. When I had been awakened and told there was a man bleeding to death in the emergency room, I hadn't taken in any of the surroundings as I raced over to the hospital. But now that nothing could be done for the patient, I continued to look around and see where I had been brought to during the night ride from El Paso.

We were surrounded by pine forests. The hospital was on a mountainside looking over a valley. The school, the tribal offices, the stores and garages were situated on the floor of the valley; the houses were scattered at random points up the mountainsides. Below the village was the White Sands Desert; above it were snow-capped Sierra Mountains. It was now about nine o'clock in the morning. The sun was already warm on my face. A woodpecker hammered away at a tree somewhere in front of the hospital.

Most Indian reservations are on badlands. San Pedro, however, was on prime land. I could see cattle grazing below in green meadows laced with mountain streams. The Apaches, under Geronimo, had kept their war against the United States going longer than any other tribe. The government had taken them more seriously and given them better land.

The undertakers came and took the body. The dead man's family and friends dispersed. The same nurse who had awakened me, led me up to the hospital kitchen to have breakfast. I was grateful she realized I hadn't eaten. As I ate by myself in a tiny dining room off the kitchen, I was thinking of my family, and how I would be phoning Lenore to tell her how beautiful San Pedro was. The cooks were talking in Apache and Dogrib. The more I listened the more it sounded like the same language. I was surprised because the two tribes lived so far apart.

I never thought about the similarity between Apache and Dogrib again until a few days later, when I was seeing an old Apache man with a pain in his belly. He spoke no English. His daughter, who spoke English and who had been serving as his translator, had stepped out of the room for a moment. He was also quite deaf. When the daughter came back, I was hovering over the old man and hollering at him:

"Eddee ayaah?"

In Dogrib that means "Where is the pain?" The old man pointed to a spot in his belly.

"Danteh?" I hollered:

In Dogrib that means: "Since when?" The old man held up one finger and said a word which sounded like *"intle"* which means "one" in Dogrib. It had been hurting him one day. The word spread instantly through the reservation: the new doctor speaks Apache.

In fact, the new doctor didn't speak Apache. He spoke very bad Dogrib. It was all just a happy coincidence. There are hundreds of Indian dialects in North America. The Apaches speak a variation of a language called Athabascan. Among the tribes that speak variations of this language are the Dogribs and Navaho. The spread of this root language has to do with early tribal migrations which link these linguistic groups to a common origin. The Apaches have an oral history which was passed down for many generations by the tribal medicine men. That history, which has now been written down, tells of a time when the Apache nation lived in "a land of eternal snow between two great lakes" —most certainly Great Slave Lake and Great Bear Lake, where the Dogribs now live. The evidence is in the language: The Dogrib word for "dog" is *"kli"*. The Apache word for "horse" is *"kli"*. These two animals serve similar hauling and transportation functions in their respective settings. When they were named, a common root word must have come to mind. All this anthropological and linguistic coincidence worked in my favour. It was the first time a doctor had arrived on the reservation "speaking" Apache.

Later that first week, I was shown a house, in the compound of houses beside the hospital, that was to be ours: it felt like anywhere and nowhere at the same time. I thought of our little house in Fort Collins. I missed the howling dogs, the little kids pulling plastic cars by a string along the snow, the scavenging ravens, and the frozen fish impaled on the stakes around the shacks. The house in the hospital compound was rent free, but I couldn't live in it.

I borrowed the hospital pick-up truck and drove up a road on the same mountain the hospital was on. After driving about ten minutes, I found a house that looked as if no one were living in it. It was half adobe and half prefab; but it really didn't matter what it was: like all the houses in San Pedro, it looked down over the valley of pine forests and the White Sands Desert in the distance, and up at the snow covered peaks of the Sierras. I drove to the next house, which was about a quarter of a mile down the road, and knocked on the door:

One of the drivers at the hospital, Franklin Jr., to whom I'd been introduced earlier in the day, answered the door. I remembered his name because of the "Jr.".

"Hi Doc, what brings you up this way?" he asked.

"I'm looking for a house to rent—"

"Why would you want to do that? There's one provided for you right beside the hospital. We've already moved furniture in there for you."

"I'd like to have more space around me—"

"I know just the place. Just a quarter of a mile down the road. It belongs to my dad—Franklin Lapaz—"

"That's what I came here to ask you about. It didn't look like anyone was living in it. I want to know if it's for rent."

"I'm sure my dad would rent it to you," Franklin Jr. answered. "One of my cousins was in it with his family for the last few years, but now they've gone to live in Santa Fe. Why don't you go down and ask him? He's just down there." Franklin Jr. pointed to a pink adobe hut in the middle of a large garden about a half a mile down the mountain.

As I drove to Franklin's house I heard a deep male voice with a slightly drunken lilt singing a song in Spanish. Beside the house was an elegant black pick-up truck with a smashed-in front end. I recognized it and remembered that I'd already met Franklin Lapaz. I had been called to help pry him out of the truck after he'd hit a tree. Franklin had been so drunk at the time that he'd barely felt the pain of four fractured ribs. The truck was new, with only thirty- five miles on it at the time of the accident.

I knocked. The singing stopped and Franklin came to the door. It opened onto the kitchen. There was a woman sitting at the table who looked drunk. There were several bottles of wine on the table: two empty and one full. Beside the wine were onions, peppers, chilis and some meat on a chopping block.

"Hi Doc, what brings you up this way?" Franklin asked. "Is this a home visit for my broken ribs?"

"No," I answered, "but how are they?"

"They're O.K.—as long as I don't breathe. Come in. I'm making some chili for supper. Why don't you join us," he said, offering me a chair at the table. "Loretta, this is the new doc who took care of me the other night when that tree came out on the road and hit me."

Loretta's gaze reminded me of the languid stare of cows as they watch you walk by their pasture fence. She was heavy and sullen, but might have been beautiful in some remote past that I was sure she couldn't remember. I nodded to her and said, "Hello"—and she nodded back lethargically.

A boy of about five or six years old was watching a cowboy movie in the living room.

"Mattie, come in and meet the new doctor," Franklin said to the boy.

I felt sorry for interrupting his TV program. "This is my son Mattie," Franklin continued. The boy managed to watch the program through the corner of his eye while we shook hands. "The doctor patched me up the night that tree got smart with me," Franklin said.

"You gotta watch it around here Mattie," I said, "Those trees can be pretty mean."

Mattie slithered happily back to the living room, and I sat down at the table.

"I'd be very happy to rent you that house," Franklin said.

He smiled at my bewilderment.

"News travels fast in San Pedro. Franklin Jr. phoned me while you were driving down here. You can have it for a hundred dollars a month. But there's one condition you have to agree to."

"What's that?" I asked.

"You have to work in our family garden every day."

"Every day?" I answered limply. "Franklin, I'd like to work in the garden. But every day? I'm a doctor. I'm busy. You know what it's like up there at the hospital—"

"I'm talking about five in the morning. It's the only time to work in a garden. Later in the day it gets too hot to work. It's our family garden. I've got two sons and a daughter. They all have children. We all work in it—and we all take whatever we need. We're all Lapaz on this mountain. You can't live here unless you become a Lapaz. Come on out. I'll show it to you."

Franklin led me out of the house and showed me his garden. It was vast and well kept. There was an elaborate system of irrigation canals running through it that I hadn't seen in any other gardens in the area.

"I bet you're wondering about that irrigation system," Franklin said.

"Yes I was," I answered, "I've never seen anything like it."

"I learned that from my father," Franklin said. "He was a Mexican prisoner in the Mexican-Apache wars. The Mexicans are much better gardeners than the Apaches. I'll show you how it works."

Suddenly Franklin left me and began running around the two acre garden and switching levers on the sluice gates of the irrigation system. After ten minutes of darting from one lever to another, he returned sweating and triumphant—and pointed to a canal twenty feet from me that was now gushing water. "That's how it works!" he panted.

"It's amazing!" I said.

He smiled and ran back over the two acres, reversing all his steps, and all his manoeuvres with the levers. By the time he returned ten minutes later—more exhausted, and sweating more, and smiling profusely—the canal twenty feet away had ceased gushing.

I was looking forward to working with Franklin at five in the morning. I guess I would have to start working on my journal at four.

Back in the house, I watched Franklin prepare the chili as he sang to himself alternately in Spanish and Apache. Loretta had fallen asleep with her head on the table, and Franklin had carried her to a couch in the living room. She was snoring loudly. This made Mattie put the volume of the TV up louder to drown out her snoring. Neither noise bothered Franklin as he cooked and sang. After chopping the vegetables, he ran out of the garden and came back with a handful of

herbs. He chopped the meat and browned it. He added the vegetables and herbs to the meat and left it on a low fire. He opened the
third bottle of wine, and poured out two glasses. "Let's drink to your
renting that house," he said.

"It's a deal," I said, raising my glass.

"Every day," he added, raising his glass.

"Every day," I added.

We drank to it.

The Prisoners' Trail

IT'S BEEN SEVERAL WEEKS now that I've been working with Franklin in
his garden every morning at five o'clock. My family is with me now
in San Pedro and we've been using the garden constantly. It's a great
garden. It has three kinds of sweet corn, including Indian corn, the
kind with kernels of three or four colours. It has the usual staples like
potatoes and tomatoes, and also has many different kinds of gourds
and beans and peppers. There are strawberry and raspberry patches,
and pumpkins and melons of several different kinds. The only thing
that was missing was anybody else working in it besides Franklin and
me.

Franklin had said it was a family garden and that all his children
and their families worked in it. Driving by the garden at other times
in the day I had sometimes seen members of his family taking vegetables from the garden, but I had never seen any of them working in
it. I noticed that the only time they would take anything from the
garden was when Franklin's truck was gone, which meant when he
wasn't around. After a few weeks of living in San Pedro, I came to
know the members of the family, and found out why I was working
alone with him. Two of his children were angry at him and weren't
talking to him. The third was the kind of a person who would take
from a garden without working in it even under the best conditions.

Franklin Jr. had only stopped talking to his father a few weeks ago.
They had been on good terms the day I stopped by Franklin Jr.'s and
asked about the house for rent. The incident that had provoked his
anger happened just before the tribal festival. Franklin Jr.'s thirteen

year old daughter was one of the girls who was participating in the puberty rite. In order for a girl to be included, their family had to donate some money for food for the feast, and provide a buckskin dancing costume for their daughter to wear in the ceremonies. The buckskin costumes cost several hundred dollars. Franklin Jr. believed that several years ago Franklin had given his other son, Desmond, the money to buy a suit for his daughter. As the festival approached, Franklin Jr. had expected Franklin would offer to buy his daughter a suit. The offer never came. As the festival drew nearer, Franklin Jr. became increasingly hurt and angry. When he was with his father he was sullen and silent. Franklin asked him why he was acting so strangely, and Franklin Jr. told him about the suit. Franklin immediately offered him the money. He explained to him that he had not paid the entire amount for Desmond, but had only given him twenty-five dollars that he was short. He explained that was why he had not thought of offering to pay for Franklin Jr.'s daughter's costume. It wasn't as if some kind of precedent had been established. It was just giving him twenty-five dollars. Frankin Jr.'s reaction was to refuse the offer, and bitterly maintain that Franklin had paid the entire amount for Desmond. As we weeded, Franklin talked forlornly about the crisis.

"Junior said to me: 'You can shove the three hundred bucks up your ass. You've always given Desmond whatever he needs without his asking. And he never does a goddamn thing for you. If I were dying of thirst in the desert, and you came by with water, I'd have to ask you for it.'"

Pausing in his weeding and reflecting for a moment, Franklin said:

"There's a lot of truth in what Junior said. Desmond always needs to be rescued. Junior is capable and looks after himself. He's always there when I need him; I never see him as needing help. But I really only did give Desmond twenty-five bucks that time for the suit. I remember he'd won the other two hundred and seventy-five playing cards. It was just a fluke that he'd come up with the money."

The daughter who wasn't talking to him had been angry for longer. That rift was about a year old. Her name was Josephine. I had come to know her well because she was a nurse with whom I worked closely in the hospital. She was the head nurse in the emergency room. I liked her very much. She was bright and had a good sense of humour. Like all Franklin's children she was striking looking. Franklin himself was one of the most handsome men I'd ever seen: he had an aquiline combination of Mayan and Apache features, softened by a charismatic and ironic smile that hovered indolently around the corners of his mouth and the lines of his face. That striking appearance was all there in Josephine and Franklin Jr.. Even Desmond had it—but in his case it was shaded by an aura of slyness, anger and weakness; he couldn't look you straight in the eye.

Josephine was tough. You had to be to run the emergency room at San Pedro. She had to handle drunks and manipulators. She had to absorb the shock of dealing with shootings and stabbings. The other day a pregnant woman was brought in who had been stabbed in the belly by another woman during a drunken brawl. The knife had gone through the unborn baby and killed it. The mother almost died as well.

Josephine had worked in the emergency room in San Pedro for seven years. She was tough, but had not been brutalized. She was still basically a kind and gentle person; she was patient and respectful with old people, and reassuring with children. Like Franklin, she was an aristocratic person who was polite with anyone whose behaviour allowed her to be so, but could adroitly handle anyone whose behaviour demanded otherwise. The first time I met Josephine she was talking to a surly Apache who was insisting on wanting his girlfriend sent to the hospital in El Paso for treatment. She had venereal warts on her vagina which were being treated adequately in San Pedro. There was no need to send her out for treatment.

"I know that her case is very serious," the man was saying, "I read her hospital chart where it said so."

"How would you get to read her chart?" countered Josephine. "The charts are confidential."

"I have my ways. I read her chart," the surly man said. He shook his finger at Josephine as he spoke. That was a mistake: "What did you read it with? That?" asked Josephine, shaking her finger at his fly which was open.

There would be one belligerent drunk or another in the emergency room every few hours who had to be dealt with. During one of my first days of working in the emergency, the receptionist came in to tell me that there was a drunk who was insisting I see him immediately but who wouldn't say why. I knew who he was. I had taken care of his wife a few days earlier. She was an alcoholic who had died of a gastrointestinal hemorrhage. She had cirrhosis of the liver. Her damaged liver had blocked her circulation and caused a fatal rupture of her esophageal veins. She had been vomiting blood and passing it through her bowel at the same time. We had transfused her with eight bottles of blood and evacuated her by helicopter to El Paso but she had died in hospital there. At the time of her death I had taken meticulous care to explain to her husband why she had died, in hope that it might lead him to stop or at least diminish his own drinking. I had tried to offer whatever solace I could, and told him to see me anytime if he felt there was anything I could do. Now here he was asking for me. Even though I was very busy with several very sick patients, I felt I should stand by my offer to see him anytime. I asked the other doctor to drop what he was doing on the ward, and take over my emergency room patients for a few moments. Actually I was glad that the husband was taking up my offer. I was gratified that even though I was new here, someone was looking towards me for some kind of support at a critical time in his life.

I took the man, whose name was Alvin, into a room, closed the door and asked him to sit down: "How are you doing, Alvin?" I asked. "It must be a rough time for you," I added.

Alvin ignored my questions and appeared to be looking straight through me, as if he barely remembered who I was, or the memory was of little consequence: "Where's her wallet?" Alvin demanded angrily.

"What?" I answered, completely dumbfounded.

"Her wallet!" He snarled menacingly. His eyes were bloodshot. It might have been partly from crying over his wife's death, but it certainly was partly from alcohol; his breath reeked of it from three feet across the table.

"What do you mean?" I asked in bewilderment.

"When she came in bleeding that day, she had a wallet in her windbreaker pocket. There was seventeen dollars in it. I've asked Josephine for it. She says they never saw a wallet. You spent a lot of time examining her. You must know where it is!"

He leaned forward menacingly and glowered at me from close up. I pulled back because at close range his breath was unbearable.

"Alvin," I said, "I don't know anything about your wife's wallet. I never saw it either. I was busy trying to save her life."

I figured I'd make a break for it now. I had to get out of sharing this small closed space with two hundred and fifty pounds of volatile belligerence. I felt like a matador pinned against the wall of the ring by an angry bull. My mistake had been in taking him alone into a room. I had to get us out of here:

"I understand the wallet was lost," I said. "I don't know anything about it. I'll bring you to the director of the hospital." I would have brought him to El Paso if he wanted. I just wanted to get out of this little space. He glowered at me without a response. I jumped up and made for the door.

I leaped into the hall. There were people in it. I could have hugged them.

"Let's go speak to the director," I said gleefully.

Alvin lumbered after me muttering: "You spent the most time with her...You were alone with her..."

The rift between Josephine and Franklin was over her mother— Franklin's ex-wife. Franklin's marriage had ended fifteen years ago when Josephine was fourteen years old. The mother was an alcoholic. For many years she had lived in Arizona with a Navaho. He died, and she drifted back to San Pedro and appeared at Josephine's door. It was the first time Josephine had seen her in ten years. She had cirrhosis of the liver. She had no money. She was depressed. Josephine took her in with her, but found it a strain on her young family. Suddenly having a depressed alcoholic stranger living among them was more than Josephine's husband and their children could bear. She appealed to Franklin for help. Franklin found a widow who was looking for someone to share her rent with. Franklin agreed to pay half the rent and a salary to the widow as a kind of keeper, and give his ex-wife money for food and clothing. Josephine had no quarrel with Franklin in terms of financial support. She felt that he had come through on that level. What horrified her was that Franklin wanted absolutely nothing to do with the woman—who after all—was her mother.

"Josephine would say to me," recounted Franklin as we weeded in the garden, "Dad, she's a sick lady. She's pathetic. It all happened fifteen years ago. You had children with her—me, for one. You can't just treat her like a stranger. And I'd say, Jo, that's what she is to me now—a stranger. And that's the way I want to leave it. I don't want to go through any of that again, I'd end up a drunk like her. I can't let that happen. I've got a young kid to take care of. That really got Jo mad—when I'd mention Mattie. Even though Josephine's a grown woman and Mattie's a little boy of six, she's jealous of him. She'd never admit it. Probably doesn't even realize it. But it's only normal. She sees me giving him the kind of care she didn't get in those years when I was squabbling with my wife."

Mattie was the boy who was watching television the night I first met Franklin. He was Franklin's son by another woman with whom he had lived for several years. They were no longer together. She was living on another reservation with another man.

Franklin had been a guide for prospectors, a goat farmer, an ambulance driver, a tribal social worker and a tribal judge. More recently he had created a tribal cattle ranch. Any tribal member could buy dollar shares. Just after the ranch came into being, the price of beef skyrocketed. The ranch prospered. It created jobs for many people. Everyone's dollar shares became worth many dollars. Franklin himself, as a major shareholder, made a large amount of money. Because of the success of the ranch, a movement arose to elect Franklin chief of the tribe at the next election. The current chief hastily pushed through the passage of a law stating that only pureblood Apaches could be eligible to run for chief. This disqualified Franklin as a candidate because of his Mexican origin.

The law had prevented Franklin from becoming the chief of the tribe, but he was its real leader. And despite the chaos of his own family life, he was everybody's father.

The fact that now both Junior and Josephine were not talking to him made Franklin very unhappy. As we worked in the garden he spoke of them both constantly:

"They're like me, both of them," Franklin would repeat. "They're proud and they're stubborn. They come by it honestly. But it will all blow over soon."

"I sure hope so," I would answer. "This is a large garden for two people to weed."

As we spoke a man in ragged clothes clutching a greasy paper bag approached the garden.

"Mornin', Dale," Franklin grunted as he pulled at a deeply rooted weed. "Did you come to help us work? The doctor here is just about to lodge a complaint with the farm labourers union about the working conditions."

"No," Dale answered with a smile. "You know me better than that, Franklin. I couldn't handle work this early in the morning. At least not until the bar opens and I've had a drink." Contradicting his statement somewhat, he leaned over and pulled at the huge root Franklin was struggling with. Dale's nose was dilated with little veins. His skin was pasty and pock-marked. There was something about his face that made you think of a fish belly—until it flashed a warm and bleary smile. The root came free and both Franklin and Dale stumbled backwards.

"I just wanted to know if you wanted to buy some light bulbs," Dale said breathlessly, as he recovered from the exertion of pulling out the root. You didn't have to be a doctor to tell he was not in great shape. He reached for the paper bag he had put down on the ground. He opened it to show us that it contained light bulbs of all different sizes. Some looked functional and some looked burnt out.

"Where are they from?" Franklin asked laughing, "My balcony and the doctor's?"

"From the chief's porch and garage, and the courthouse," Dale said with a smile. "And there's insect repellent bulbs from the baptist minister and the parole officer."

"You've been busy," Franklin said laughing, "but I don't need any light bulbs. I do need some help with this garden or the doctor's going to quit. I'll pay you five dollars an hour to do some weeding. That's a dollar above minimum wage. And I'll advance you two bucks to buy a drink." Franklin took two dollars out of his pocket and gave it to Dale. "Go have a drink when the bar opens at eight and come back ready to work."

Dale snapped up the two dollars and put it in his pocket. He closed the bag of light bulbs and smiled. "Be back at eight-fifteen," he said. "Unless I can sell some of these to the bartender. Then I might be a little longer. Maybe nine or so. Thanks Franklin. Bye, Doc. Don't work too hard."

We could see Dale moving along the path to the tribal bar which was just at the foot of the mountain. "Will he come back to weed?" I asked.

"Not in a million years," Franklin said, pausing for a moment and leaning on a hoe. "He was once one of the best cowboys the tribal ranch ever had. He did well on the rodeo circuit for a while. He'll be back another morning. But not to weed. He'll have some towels or shirts to sell that he's stolen from somebody's clothesline. He was once a reliable worker. Now he's just a drunk on the Prisoners' Trail. Here Doc, help me with this weed," he said, suddenly pointing to a large thick weed that could take two people to give it a good yank. I knew that he had suddenly turned his attention to it because thinking about Dale made him sad and he wanted to get him off his mind.

The Prisoners' Trail is a path that makes a circle around the out-skirts of the reservation and heads across the county line. It's a vaga-bond trail for outlaws wanted by the tribal police for minor offences. There was an unwritten understanding that the police wouldn't arrest anyone who was on the Prisoners' Trail if their crime was truly minor. It was a kind of unofficial no-man's-land. A minor charge was usually dropped after a month. The Trail was a practical outdoor jail. Its path ran by both Franklin's house and mine.

The Trail people were enthusiastic users of Franklin's garden. They also made regular visits to my chicken house. They confined them-selves to eggs and never stole chickens. I don't think the chickens were spared out of politeness. I think it was just too much hassle to kill one and cook it. Most of the people who staggered along the trail were not domestically inclined.

Later on that same morning that Dale had come by with the bag of light bulbs, I was driving to the hospital and passed a point where the Prisoners' Trail intersects with the main highway. There was a crowd of people milling around a body covered with a sheet. One of the tribal policemen flagged me down.

"We were just going to call you to pronounce this man dead," the policeman said. He was struck by a car. Hit and run."

I lifted the sheet to see Dale's fish-belly, pock-marked face. There was no transforming smile. A few feet from the body was a torn paper bag and some broken light bulbs.

"He was once one of our best cowboys," the policeman said.

Home

THE POLICEMAN who had uttered Dale's eulogy at the roadside was a mild-mannered and sensitive Zuni Indian named Carlos Three Star. The department of Indian Affairs had a policy of policing reservations with Indians from other tribes. The reason that the department of Indian Affairs offered for this practice was that it "allowed the police to function free of the influence of family and friends."

These policemen from another tribe were resented, and of course felt alienated. The net result was a mean police force. The police would often bring in prisoners from the jail to the hospital with large open cuts on their head which required stitching. These cuts were clearly blackjack wounds, but the police would say, "They slipped and hit their head."

A prime example of one of these alienated policemen was Cloud Eagle, a burly six-foot-four Sioux Indian who called me on a Sunday afternoon about twelve o'clock and said:

"Hello, Doc, have you had your lunch yet?"

"No, I haven't," I answered.

"That's good," he said.

"Why's that?" I asked.

"Well, if you'd had it, you might have found it hard to keep it down when you get here to house number thirty-eight on Nogal Canyon Road. There's been a double shooting. We've already called for an ambulance. You'd better get here fast."

At house number thirty-eight a man had shot his wife in the belly and then shot himself in the head. His wife was still alive. I put an intravenous needle in her forearm to pump in fluid to try and replace the blood she was losing. A rifle was draped across the dead man's chest. The nozzle of the gun pointed to a pulpy, bloody torn lump of flesh at the end of his neck that had once been his face. There were several children wandering around the house crying. Someone was trying to comfort them. We placed the woman in the ambulance and sped towards the Air Force Hospital in Almagordo. She had a cardiac arrest ten minutes from the hospital. I was unable to resuscitate her, nor was a team which took over on our arrival at the hospital and tried for an hour.

Carlos Three Star, the policeman who had pronounced Dale's eulogy at the roadside, was one policeman who succeeded in not relating to the tribe as an outsider. He had an inherent respect for other people which led him to treat everyone as fairly as he could. He tried to make life easier rather than harder for prisoners in his care. The Apaches responded by treating him as if he were one of their own. That was why Carlos would say of Dale:

"He was one of our best cowboys."

Carlos's wife Juanita was a nurse at the hospital. She was just like him. Her relation to other people was guided by genuine respect for just about everyone's essential worth. I said just about everyone, because I guess that even for Juanita there were some people that fall below certain limits we all define for ourselves. Anyway, enough philosophy. Back to Carlos and Juanita. To put it simply: they were always there for everybody, and consequently almost everyone was always there for them. Again, I say almost everyone because as you've probably noticed, there are some people who can take and not give. But I said I wouldn't get philosophical, so back to Carlos and Juanita. It was typical of them that when we first arrived in San Pedro Juanita was the only person to invite us to her home, and take the time and consideration to show us around the reservation and the neighbouring towns. Her invitation came at a moment when we were feeling stranded.

Carlos and Juanita had one four year old child. He had been left crippled in infancy by meningitis, an infection of the membranes surrounding the spinal cord. After several years of trying unsuccessfully to have another child, Juanita became pregnant. She was determined that nothing would go wrong. She approached me early in the pregnancy and said:

"I'm pregnant. About three weeks now. Would you deliver my baby?"

"I'd like to very much," I answered.

"But I'm going to ask you to promise one thing which I know is difficult for you," she added.

"What's that?" I asked.

"As a nurse I hate to ask you this. I understand how important it is to have time off. But I want you to promise that even if you're not on call when I go into labour that you'll come in and do the delivery."

"It's a promise," I answered.

Juanita's labour did become complicated. Juanita was tiny. Either her baby was too large for her to deliver vaginally, or it was in a position that would require the help of an obstetrician to turn it with forceps if it didn't turn on its own. I called for an ambulance to take her to the hospital at the airforce base thirty miles away in Almagordo. If her labour improved on its own, and she delivered along the way in the ambulance, that would be a happy outcome. On the other hand, if her labour didn't improve, I was certainly going to need the help of an obstetrician, either for a rotation of the baby with forceps or a delivery by caesarean section.

When I had looked at the ambulance driver schedule, I had seen that a driver named Charley was on call. When the ambulance pulled up to the evacuation area, I was surprised to find Franklin Jr. was driving: "How come you're driving, Franklin?" I asked.

"As soon as she got pregnant Juanita made me promise that if she had to be evacuated during her labour, I would drive whether I was on call or not," Franklin said, and added "I notice you're not supposed to be working today either."

We sped across the desert with the accelerator pushed to the floor. Against the desert's sparse background the speed was almost imperceptible. It was only when we flashed by the occasional passing car that our speed became evident. Carlos sat in the front beside Franklin, and I sat in the back beside Juanita's stretcher. As we inched across the vast desert in this little box on wheels, the new life in Juanita's belly declared itself in heartbeats we could hear amplified on the fetal monitor. Her contractions were now coming every two to three minutes and lasting a minute. She was in pain but barely expressed it. She would grimace during contractions but hardly uttered a sound.

When we reached Almagordo, Franklin put on the siren and weaved deftly through the cars that were scurrying out of the way. Juanita had her baby six hours after we arrived in Almagordo. She had continued to have a slow and difficult labour. The baby was much larger than her first child, and was in a position that required a rotation with forceps by an obstetrician. I expected him to say that he wasn't really on call, but Juanita had spoken to him eight months ago, and made him promise that if she needed a forceps rotation or caesarean section that he would come in to do it. After applying the forceps and turning the baby, he insisted, out of courtesy, that I complete the delivery. It was a girl. The labour had been long and complicated, but the baby showed no signs of any complications. She was breathing well and crying vigorously. Her reflexes and movements were brisk. Her colour was good. I guess she had promised Juanita to be born in perfect condition. Carlos stayed with Juanita in Almagordo and Franklin Jr. and I drove home in the ambulance at normal speed. Now it really felt like we were crawling across the desert. Franklin and I were hungry. It had been ten hours since we'd eaten. We stopped at a restaurant on the outskirts of Almagordo. While we were eating, the phone behind the lunch counter rang. The one waitress in the place answered. The restaurant was very small and she was a very loud woman. Every word she uttered was forced on everyone's attention;

…"You're looking for who?" she hollered into the phone.

"Elvin Harris? No I don't know anyone by that name…How old?…He's confused and he slobbers saliva on himself…walks unsteady…Wait. Hold on a minute."

She lay the phone down beside the receiver and headed for an elderly man sitting alone at a table. He was eating soup. His hand quivered slightly each time he brought it to his mouth.

"You Elvin Harris?" the waitress asked the old man.

"Not yet," the old man answered.

By the time we got back to San Pedro I had fallen asleep in the ambulance. Juanita's labour had begun fifty-two hours earlier and all I'd had were scattered moments of sleep like these. I woke to Franklin gently shaking me as we pulled into the hospital garage.

"Hey Doc, we're home," he said.

Clifford's Boots

IN AUTUMN, if the tribal game wardens judge that elk is plentiful, the San Pedro Apaches hold an elk hunt. Lots are drawn and a small number of tribal members win the right to kill a buck. Hunting groups of family and friends form around a winning ticket holder.

The hunt is conducted on horseback, as horses are needed to haul the slain and quartered elk out of the woods. Franklin Jr., who knew I couldn't shoot or ride, invited me to become part of his group.

"You know I can't shoot or ride, Franklin," I said. "I'd just be a nuisance."

"Don't worry," Franklin Jr. said, "we'll teach you."

Because of the heavy load of work we always had at the hospital, plans I had made to learn something about riding and shooting had come to nothing by the day of the hunt. I hadn't even had time to buy a rifle. Franklin Jr. took Lenore into town and selected a deer rifle which she bought for me.

During the three days of the hunt everyone in the hunting party tried to teach me how to ride and shoot. But one man in his early twenties named Clifford, especially took it upon himself to stick by my side and correct every mistake I made. He was always there offering criticism and encouragement at critical moments: "Doc, you're getting on the wrong side of the horse again," Clifford might say, or "Doc, put that gun back on safety! If you stumble, you'll go to the moon!"

Though several of the men were twice Clifford's age, he was by far the best hunter and woodsman. Most of the older men had become heavy and slow moving. Clifford was lean and wiry and moved quickly. It was no surprise that it was Clifford who shot our party's buck. It happened on the evening of the second day out. We were camped on a mountain top. There was only one day of the hunt left. A few deer had been sighted, but no elk. It was dusk, and we were sitting around a campfire talking while supper was cooking. Suddenly the sound of antlers colliding, and an angry bellowing were heard from another mountain top, about three or four miles away. The elk could be seen with field glasses. Two bulls were fighting in a clearing, and a herd of cows were grazing off in the woods beside them.

The older men assured one another that by the time anyone got over there it would be too dark to shoot. While they were talking, Clifford slipped out unnoticed.

An hour later, just as night was falling, a shot rang out from the other mountain top. Another hour later, Clifford came back—sweating, exhausted, and elated. He'd shot a buck.

The next morning, Clifford led us up the other mountain to where his buck lay. The men skinned it, quartered it, and loaded the quarters on the horses. Because the sight of blood panics the horses, the men blindfold them while the meat is being loaded on them. Even the smell of blood sets the horses rearing and whinnying as the elk quarters are draped over their saddles and tied to the saddle horns.

On the trip down the mountain, when we had stopped by a stream for water, Clifford moved up beside me and put his hand on my shoulder. He pointed to a thicket across the stream about seventy yards away. I saw nothing but a thicket.

"Pick up your rifle!" he whispered.

Twenty seconds later, a whitetail deer pranced out from behind the brush.

"Now!" Clifford whispered again.

My hands shook. The bullet whirred off somewhere beside the deer, and both disappeared into the thicket.

"When we get back, I'll take you to the target practice," Clifford said.

I went to the target practice myself for several months.

One Sunday morning, about four months after the elk hunt, I was returning from feeding our chickens, when I saw Clifford coming up the hill to our house. He was coming from behind the house, where there was nothing but miles of meadow and brush. It was the first time anyone had ever come from that direction. Everyone else had come from the road in front of the house. I hadn't seen him since the elk hunt.

"Get your rifle, Doc," he said, "we gotta practice."

Clifford had worked for several years as a medical technician in the hospital, but had been fired for hitting one of the doctors. It had happened before I began working there. About the incident Clifford says: "The doctor was being rude to an old Apache, so I had to hit him."

His training as a medical technician had taken several years, and included two years at a technical school off the reservation. But his qualifications were only recognized within the Indian Health Service, and they refused to rehire him. Since he had been fired, he worked as hunting guide for white hunters. The work was only occasional. He spent much of his time alone in a tent in the woods. He drank heavily and continually. It was rare that he was not at least slightly drunk.

At the target practice, mostly because he was fairly drunk, and partly because I had improved my aim, I outshot Clifford. He was delighted. He was immensely proud of me. Quite correctly, he considered himself responsible. In my months of solitary practice, I had been guided entirely by what he showed me on the three days of the elk hunt. He carefully took down the two targets, folded them and put them into his pocket.

"I'm going to show everyone the Doc outshot me," he drawled happily.

Clifford spent the rest of the day at our house. After showing the targets to Lenore and Mark, my five year old son, he showed them to everyone who came by that day:

"The Doc outshot me," he'd say. "That's his target, and that's mine."

One of the people who came by was a British doctor who was considering applying for work in San Pedro. The other doctor in our two-man hospital was leaving in six months, and his position had been advertised. The British doctor was working his way around the globe. He had stopped by my house to sound me out about the job. He had an arrogant air about him. It was clear that he felt he was in "the colonies." He had an American girl with him. She was very quiet. She was probably feeling the bewilderment most Americans or Canadians feel the first time they are on a reservation. It is America or Canada; and yet it's not. It's somewhere else: somewhere Oriental and prehistoric—somewhere initially threatening.

By this time, we had been joined by Josephine and her husband Bruce with their children who had come by for a Sunday visit, and Franklin Jr. and his wife who had seen Josephine's truck in front of our house, and had come over with their children. Franklin Jr. and Bruce had brought beer and Clifford drank most of it. The more he drank, the more clear it became that he didn't like the British doctor. Clifford had spent two years in Albuquerque during his training as a technician. He had once lived in Los Angeles for a year. When he met an arrogant white man like the British doctor, he would play the role of the inarticulate savage, the primitive Indian who had never left the reservation. He showed the doctor and his girl the targets: "The Doc outshot me. That's his. That's mine," he said, weaving precariously over them, with the targets in one hand, and a bottle in the other.

"Yes, rather remarkable," muttered the doctor.

The doctor was annoyed. None of the Apaches, except Clifford who was drunk and clearly hostile, had acknowledged his presence or expressed any interest in him. No one had encouraged him to work here. He found vent for his anger in a question ostensibly directed to me, but meant for Clifford: "Why do Indians have such an alcohol problem?" the doctor asked.

Clifford put his bottle down on the table and answered: "It's not a problem, Mr. Doctor." Clifford lifted his bottle from the table and took a long guzzle, all the while leaning toward the doctor and looking at him straight in the eye: "We just like to drink—that's all," he said.

The doctor left five minutes later. He never came back.

Clifford continued to drop by sporadically. I tried to get him back his job at the hospital but never succeeded. One night he came by looking particularly dejected. He had taken a job as a bartender in a hotel the tribe maintained for tourists. Despite his drinking, he'd always had a characteristic equanimity and poise. Both were shattered. He had felt a certain kind of pride in working as a hunting guide, but there wasn't enough work available. He found working as a bartender among the tourists demeaning. A few minutes after he arrived, I was called down to the hospital to deliver a baby. I left Clifford in the living room with Mark, our five year old. Lenore had fallen asleep beside Allen, our two year old, when she was putting him to bed. When I left, Mark was showing Clifford how to gamble with a dredyl, a top with four Hebrew letters engraved on it. You spin it and bet on which letter it will land on. Within seconds Clifford perfected the pronunciation of the Hebrew letters. When I returned three hours later, at one in the morning, they were still playing. Their piles of pennies were about even. There was also a pile of empty beer bottles beside Clifford. He had brought them in from his car. By now he was very drunk. They were both laughing uproariously and having a great time.

I put Mark to sleep. Clifford went for the living room couch and fell asleep. I roused him, and told him I'd drive him to his brother Willard's, a tribal medicine man, who lived about a mile away. I didn't want to wake the family in the morning and have to deal with Clifford with a hangover. The time spent together at breakfast with the family was often the only time I would see them until late at night. I led Clifford to the car.

A week later, about nine o'clock at night, I had a call from the other doctor:

"I knew you'd want to know," he said solemnly. "Clifford Enjady was just killed in his car. He drove off that deep gulley near the Inn. He was on the way home from work. He was comatose when I got there. It was probably an intracerebral bleed. I intubated him, and thought we might make it down to Almagordo, but he was dead by the time we got to Tularosa."

A priest who hadn't known Clifford droned his way through the church service. A wax doll Clifford dressed in a three piece suit and a polka-dot tie and stick pin, lay displayed in the coffin. It was the first time I'd ever seen him without his cowboy hat on. His hair was plastered down with grease and parted in the center.

After the priest had mumbled the last graveside prayer, the funeral really began. Willard had been standing beside the priest. He suddenly wheeled around and turned his back on Clifford's grave. Placing his hands on his hips, and looking up defiantly at the sky, he said in Apache: "My brother liked to drink. He died happy."

From a bag that had been lying beside him, Willard took out Clifford's cowboy boots and hunting knife. He cut long slashes in the soles of each boot, and placed them in the grave. The slashed boots would discourage Clifford's spirit from walking about and haunting the living. He placed Clifford's knife and his old brown cowboy hat in the grave beside the boots. He followed it with Clifford's deer rifle and his saddle, and then stepped back. Relatives and friends walked up to the grave and threw in blankets, jewelry and ammunition. When the offerings were over, his closest male friends and relatives took turns shovelling earth into the grave. I stood in the back, among the few white people who were there. Willard made his way toward me and handed me a shovel.

I stepped forward and shovelled some earth into the grave. As the pebbles rattled across the coffin lid, I thought of the night, a week ago, when I'd turned Clifford out of my house. Suddenly, I appreciated the wisdom in slashing Clifford's boots. Willard had done a very complete job. I suppose he had reasons of his own for being so thorough.

The Rattlesnake

LENORE LOOKED OUT our front window and saw a diamond-patterned clump in the bushes just where Mark was waiting for the bus that takes him to kindergarten. She noticed it just as he entered safely on the bus and the doors closed behind him. She ran to the phone and called me at the hospital:

"I think there's a rattlesnake in the bushes just where Mark gets on the bus!" she said. "Maybe the snake has a nest there or something, because he's not moving! He's just staying there."

I drove immediately to Franklin's. He was having breakfast. Franklin Jr. and Desmond were with him. "Franklin, I need your help", I said. "Lenore thinks she sees a rattlesnake hanging out where the school bus stops for Mark."

"If she's right we better get rid of it," Franklin said, rising immediately from his seat.

"I'm sorry to disturb your breakfast," I said, as Franklin took a shotgun from a gun rack on his wall and loaded the magazine with shells.

"My breakfast will be there when I come back," Franklin said. "The snake may leave and come back sometime when Mark's there. It may have a nest around there."

Franklin Jr. and Desmond followed Franklin into his truck. I went over to the truck to tell Franklin where the bush was. Franklin was driving. Franklin Jr. sat beside him and Desmond sat over by the other window. As we spoke I was struck by the same profile on the three faces in a line. Beside Franklin were two powerful men with his features. These two men who resembled him also loved him, respected him and were loyal to him. They had a very tight army to face the world with. I thought of my own two little boys sitting beside me. Someday when they were grown men, I wondered if I would be worthy of the kind of respect that Franklin had from his sons. Franklin had taught his sons how to fish and hunt and garden. He had taught them how to tend cattle, cut wood, mend fences, and fix broken windows and water pipes. He had taught them how to use a compass and how to change a tire.

I couldn't think of anything specific that I've ever taught either of my sons except a few things I've learned from books. I had been brought up in a North American ghetto where all I was expected to learn was in books, and where my father felt his only role in what I had to learn was to provide the money to pay for my education. As a result my only tangible knowledge was medicine. I can't really teach my boys medicine, but I hope that the way I try to practice it is teaching them something about respecting other human beings. That's a very abstract heritage. It doesn't provide food or warmth or shelter. It leaves you very dependent on others, and defenceless if they turn on you. It has about as much survival value as Dale's light bulbs after they were shattered on the road. If you consider the history of man to date, there's certainly no viable argument for living at other people's mercy. As a matter of fact, when you think about it, it's a very crazy thing to do.

Since the elk hunt I had taught myself to shoot, but I would never trust myself to hit a snake from a distance, and run the risk of missing it and have it return to haunt that corner. So once again, for survival I was dependent on someone else. I can't fix anything. Whenever I try to fix something, I make it worse. In the end I have to pay somebody more when I finally hire them to fix it. Or I mangle it so much that no one can fix it, and I have to buy a new one. I can't even fix a leaking faucet.

Driving from Franklin's house to mine on this sunlit morning in New Mexico, I felt like an aged European Jew in a long frock coat and fedora: a wandering Jew with no land, and with none of the skills that landowners cherish and pass on to their young. Here I was again, as so many times before, bartering cerebration for physical service. There is nothing I can do about it. I'm too old to change. It's my heritage. Whoever heard of a Jew killing a rattlesnake?

I arrived at the corner before they did. They had stopped at Franklin Jr.'s for his gun. The plan was for Franklin Jr. to take the first shot. His father would be ready to take a second shot if he missed. I parked about fifty yards away. I peered at the bush near the bus stop and saw the diamond-patterned spot among the leaves that Lenore had described.

Franklin and his sons arrived. They knelt with the two guns in firing position. Franklin Jr.'s first shot shattered the diamond- patterned spot. I joined Franklin and his sons as they advanced on the bush. Franklin thrust a stick into the bush and emerged with the remnants of a diamond-patterned bandana—the kind a cowboy might wear around his neck.

"There's your rattlesnake, Doc," Franklin said. "Let's go show it to Lenore."

The story of the rattlesnake circulated quickly around the village. Men would smile when they saw me coming. They would point to diamond-patterned bandanas and say: "Watch out, Doc. It bites!"

One of These Days

YOU MAY HAVE NOTICED when Franklin and his sons were shooting the diamond-patterned bandana that Franklin Jr. was talking to his father again. I was very happy about that. Not just because I liked them both and knew it was causing them both pain, but because Franklin Jr. started helping in the garden. Josephine was also talking to Franklin. Again, I was happy for both of them. I was also delighted because Josephine's husband Bruce showed up regularly for weeding. There seemed to be a whole family renaissance. Even Desmond who was a heavy drinker, gambler and man-about-town was showing up now and then.

We had become part of the Lapaz family. Franklin was our patriarch as well as theirs. We had become one extended family. However, the period of complete harmony didn't last long. Soon Josephine and I weren't talking to each other—except professionally in the hospital when we had to. The rift between Josephine and me occurred in the second year we were in San Pedro. It happened at the time of the tribal feast. Once again the population swelled from two thousand to well over ten thousand, with the same logarithmic explosion of sickness, accidents, births and deaths. It was a Saturday afternoon. I had stopped by the hospital for a moment to pick up some mail. Mark was with me. As I sorted through the mail and Mark constructed a chain of paper clips, suddenly a wailing woman carrying a dead baby appeared at the door of my office accompanied by a crowd of people. Mark saw the dead baby and turned pale. I had to get him out of there but I couldn't leave. I had to deal with the mother. All of a sudden I saw Josephine going by in the hallway outside my office. I called her in and took her aside.

"Jo," I said desperately, "you see what's happening here—you've got to get Mark out of here for me. Please take him home right away, o.k.?"

"Sorry, I can't," Josephine answered.

"Why not?" I asked.

"I've got my mother with me. She's already impatient to get to the feast grounds."

"It would only take you ten minutes. This is too much for a six year old to deal with. Supposing she gets to the feast ten minutes later."

"She's already very grumpy today. I was just coming here to pick up her anti-depressant—"

"Just forget it," I interrupted, and turned my attention back to the wailing mother. I didn't want to hear about Josephine's mother's twenty-year depression at this point. I put Mark out in the hallway in a chair.

The people with the baby were Navahos. Several of them were drunk and reeked of alcohol. The mother's face was contorted with grief and her body was shaking as she sobbed: "I went to feed him," she wailed, "and found him dead."

"Had he been sick?"

"No."

"No cough?…vomiting?…diarrhea?…fever?"

"No, nothing."

"How old is he?"

"Two months."

"Was there any trouble when he was born?"

"No."

Examination of the baby didn't offer any clues to why he died. Two families who had come for the feast were sharing a van. There were about twelve people sleeping on the floor of the van in sleeping bags. Someone might have fallen asleep in a drunken stupor and rolled on the baby and suffocated him. Then again, it could have been a case of Sudden Infant Death Syndrome, when a baby suddenly stops breathing for reasons that no one has yet been able to explain. There was nothing more I could do. I tried to comfort the mother. She didn't know me or trust me. My efforts became an interference in her mourning. The father was back in Arizona. I phoned the social service worker on call to help the family make arrangements to get the baby's body back to their reservation in Arizona for burial. There was nothing more I could do. Now I could take Mark home. I went out to the hall to find Mark still stunned by the sight of the dead baby and full of questions about him.

Josephine had let me down. I couldn't see how she wouldn't have wanted to help me at that moment. I couldn't see how getting to the feast ten minutes later could balance against sparing a six-year old from being witness to that kind of horror. Two months went by and Josephine and I hadn't spoken to each other, except professionally in the hospital. It was a shame because our two families had gotten on well. Lenore and Josephine had become friends, and I had become friends with her husband Bruce. He was a Pueblo Indian Josephine had met when he had come as a visitor to the tribal feast. Just before the quarrel between Josephine and I had occurred, Bruce had taken us to his pueblo near Taos to visit with his family. Bruce had a job on the tribal forestry crew, and was taking courses at night in a nearby college from which he would eventually graduate as a case worker in juvenile deliquency. Since the incident we missed sitting around talking to them.

One Sunday afternoon Josephine phoned me because her fourteen-month-old baby Suzanna was ill. I knew she knew I was not the doctor on call that day:

"When did it start?" I asked.

"Just this morning," she answered.

"Are there any other symptoms?"

"No. That's what worries me. If there were something straightforward like a cough or diarrhea or vomiting, I'd feel more at ease."

"I'll come over there and examine her. If we need to get a blood count or a culture we'll go down to the hospital."

Walking over to Josephine's I figured it was time to forget about what had happened that time. She had felt that I was asking her to put my son over her mother. I would just forget it. I also understood why she was calling me even though I wasn't on call. The doctor on call was a new doctor who was also the new director of the hospital. The reason Josephine had called me, even though we weren't talking, was because the new doctor was incompetent. It was a big problem. I might have let him treat some of my old political enemies from Fort Collins, but I wouldn't have let him treat Josephine's baby. Josephine wasn't an enemy. She was a friend who had disappointed me. And now that was all over anyway—and I was glad it was. Come to think of it, I wouldn't even let him treat an enemy's baby.

When I arrived at Josephine and Bruce's house it was clear to all of us that everything was back to normal in our relation. Her calling and my coming said it all: "Hi, Jo. Hi, Bruce," I said.

"Hi, Doc. Thanks for coming over," Bruce said.

Suzanna was on a blanket on the living room floor. She looked ill. She had none of her usual lustre. She was usually a very busy baby with big black eyes that were always taking in everything that was happening. She was always luring everybody around her into playing with her. Now she lay there disinterested. It was not just because of her fever. Infants can have high fevers with simple colds and still be alert and active. She was ill.

Josephine watched tensely as I examined Suzanna. She knew exactly what I was hoping to find and what I was hoping not to find. I wanted to find an infected ear drum or inflamed tonsils with pus on them—something relatively minor and easily treated. I couldn't find either of those —or anything else minor. What I did find was what we were hoping I wouldn't find: something major. Her neck was stiff. Josephine watched as I tried to gently flex Suzanna's neck and met with stiffness and an irritable high-pitched cry.

"Jo, I think you know what I'm thinking," I said.

"Meningitis?" Josephine questioned, her voice quavering and not sounding like her own.

"Looks enough like it that we've got to do an L.P. right away," I answered. "Let's go down to the hospital."

Josephine wrapped Suzanna in a blanket and took her in her arms. "Let's go." she said.

L.P. stands for lumbar puncture. When you suspect meningitis you put a needle into the spinal canal and draw off spinal fluid for analysis. The spot for penetration of the canal is in the lumbar or lower back area, because the vertebrae are larger there and have proportionally more space between. Meningitis in an infection of the membranes enclosing the brain and the spinal cord. It can cripple, cause mental retardation and kill. The sooner it is diagnosed and treatment begun the less likely it is that complications will occur. Treatment is at least two weeks of intravenous antibiotic. With babies it means tying them down to a bed. It's not a treatment you're going to begin without clear evidence. The evidence is in the spinal fluid. When you draw it out with a needle you may see obvious pus in it if the infection is advanced. When you put the fluid under a microscope you see inflammatory cells if the fluid is infected. Chemical analysis of the fluid will show an increase in protein and decrease in sugar if infection is present. After these initial observations, you put a few drops of the fluid away for incubation, and within a day you know which bacteria is causing the disease and which antibiotics it's sensitive to. You begin treatment with intravenous antibiotic the moment you have spinal fluid with evidence of infection. Getting spinal fluid from between the lumbar vertebrae of a squirming baby depends a lot on how well the baby is held by the nurse or orderly helping you. They have to hold the baby with its head jack- knifed tightly against its knees. Josephine had assisted me on other cases and had done very well. I made the mistake of asking her to hold Suzanna. When I found my spot between the vertebrae and inserted the needle, Josephine faltered and relaxed her hold. Suzanna moved. I missed the spot. I obtained fluid but there was blood in it. It would still give us the bacteriological evidence the next day, but the blood made initial diagnosis impossible. Cells, sugar and protein from the blood would confound the analysis. I asked another nurse to hold Suzanna. I tried again at a point about an inch higher up on the spinal cord. The vertebrae higher up are smaller, and the space between them smaller. I found it harder to find a spot that I was confident about. I missed a second time. Once again there was blood in the fluid.

I put the spinal fluid into an incubator, and began treating Suzanna. We tied her down to a bed and put an intravenous needle in her scalp. We would only know the next day if the diagnosis was right. Because meningitis is so serious, we send the patients to a pediatric ward in El Paso for the two weeks of treatment, so that they are among relevant specialists if complications arise. Suzanna and Josephine left by ambulance.

The next day bacteriological culture confirmed the diagnosis. Suzanna had meningitis. The bacteria causing the illness was sensitive to the antibiotic she was receiving. There was every expectation she would do well. And she did. Within a few weeks she was the same old busy baby with large black eyes, taking in everything and luring everyone into playing with her.

When Suzanna recovered completely Franklin made a chili supper for all of us. I knew he was also doing it because he was glad that Josephine and I had patched up our quarrel. Franklin got fairly drunk at the meal, so it didn't surprise me when he came to my door at five in the morning with a bellyache. I examined him and figured it was a gastritis from alcohol. I drove down to the hospital and got him some antacid. He took it home with him but was no better in the morning. I won't go into the whole diagnostic story, but, in short, within a few days Franklin was in hospital in El Paso with cancer of the stomach. At operation it was found to be a localized lesion. That means it wasn't widespread. They were able to remove the tumour and leave part of his stomach. Cancer of the stomach is a tumour with a bad reputation for recurrence. If you make it for five years without recurrence you're probably cured. But only about thirty percent of patients last the five years.

While Franklin was in hospital in El Paso we kept Mattie with us.

Mattie's kind of a loner — Franklin's all he has. Without him he's lost. We tried to bring him into our family life but with little response. Mark sometimes succeeded in getting him to play, but he was in a daze. At one point when I put him on the phone to speak to Franklin he said: "What do the doctors say, Daddy?...Is it cancer?"

I was stunned. I hadn't imagined that he even knew the word. Franklin was his whole family. He knew that he could lose his whole family at once. No wonder he was dazed.

Franklin himself understood clearly the seriousness of his disease. I went to see him in El Paso before the operation. He had smiled ironically and said: "Doc, if this thing is advanced and I die from it over the next while, I want you to tell everyone I don't want a big funeral. Tell them to put me in a gunnysack and throw me over an arroyo."

"Franklin, nobody's going to be thinking about your remains for a long time," I answered. "I'm sure it's going to be a small growth that they can remove easily, and that'll be the last we ever hear from it."

I wish I could do as good a job on his stomach cancer as he and his sons did on that diamond-patterned bandana.

The Fender-jack

THE FRENZIED DIRECTOR of the hospital, who had picked me up at the airport the night I had first arrived in San Pedro, had been fired several days after I met him. He was one of a string of directors who had not been able to survive being caught in the middle of the battles between the tribe and the government. Over the next two years there were several more who came and left. Some were fired and some quit. The latest director was a middle-aged doctor from Kansas. It was the first time a doctor had been given the job. The plan was for him to do administrative work half-time and work as a doctor the other half. It might have worked were he not incompetent medically. He also seemed to be on the lam. Every time the phone rang he looked apprehensive. I didn't know for sure that he was running from something, but I did know for certain that he was an incompetent doctor. There were several incidents where he almost killed people.

The only thing that saved them was good luck; they'll never know how close they came. That was why Josephine had called me that Sunday afternoon when Suzanna was ill and the new director was on call.

I phoned the regional director to tell him about the problem. I explained that the new director was medically incompetent and dangerous: "He's going to kill someone," I said.

"You should be trying to help him instead of complaining about him," the regional director answered. "Perhaps his hospital skills are weak after years of office practice. But he has a maturity that you and your other younger colleague lack."

"He's going to kill someone," I said.

"I'm sure that's just an alarmist view of the situation," the regional director answered. "Put your energy into helping him instead of tattling on him."

I phoned the national director in Washington. I was told he would be unavailable for several weeks and was transferred to one of his administrative assistants. I told the assistant about the director's lethal medical care. It was like talking to a recorded message. I put down the phone feeling assured that every word I said would be used against me until such time as I was assassinated.

One day several weeks later the state police drove up and took the new director away. Fortunately he was wanted for fraud in Kansas. Everyone breathed a sigh of relief. The tribal council asked if I were willing to be director of the hospital. They said they would ask the government to appoint me. I was moved by the offer but had to say no. I explained that I had commitments that were drawing me back to Canada, and that I was just about to tell the government that I intended to leave within the next few months.

I had no commitments in Canada; in fact I didn't know where we were going next. All I knew was that we had to leave by autumn when Mark would be school age. For us it was a sad fact that the elementary school in San Pedro didn't have a level of education that we knew he could have back in Canada. Even if we struggled to supplement it ourselves with the little time we had, I had seen that the few white children who went to the school were often teased mercilessly by the Apache children. I didn't want to tell the tribal council the real reason, but there was no way we could stay in San Pedro.

A week later I received a letter from the tribal council. It was an invitation to a feast the tribe was making in honour of our family in appreciation of "our contribution to tribal life" over the time we had been there. I thought that was a generous response after I had declined the offer to be director and had announced I was leaving. It was going to be hard to go.

Everything we were taking with us was in our pick-up truck. The rest of our things would be sent by moving van when we had a house to send it to. Franklin had been helping me pack. Now that we were finished packing and were about to leave, he turned to me and said: "I hear they have some pretty deep snow in Canada."

"That's true," I said, without really thinking about Franklin's statement or why he might be making it. My mind was on packing and trying to make sure about what to take with us now and what to leave for the moving van.

"What would you do if you were out driving in a snowstorm and you had a flat?" Franklin asked.

"I would change the tire," I answered. It was a complete bluff. I'm Jewish. I'd never changed a flat tire in my life.

"Show me your jack," Franklin said.

I'd never looked at the jack that came with the truck. There was a panel near the back wheel that housed it. I opened the panel and took out the jack. I'd never changed a tire, but even I could tell the jack looked small. "That's the jack they give you with this truck," Franklin said. "What do you think of it?"

"It looks kind of small," I answered. "Sort of like a can-opener."

"That's about how useful you'll find it," Franklin said. "Just think of yourself lying in the snow under the truck trying to lift it with a small jack like that. The first gust of wind would knock the truck down right on top of you."

"It all sounds pretty terrible. I don't think I'm going to go back to Canada after all—"

"I'm serious, Doc," Franklin said. "What would you do?"

"I'd call you long distance—"

"Here's what you'd do," Franklin said. He went over to his truck. On the back wall of the cab was a wire screen on which Franklin kept his essential tools. Most of the men in San Pedro had a screen like this on their truck on which they hung a shovel, an ax, a gun rack and a fender-jack. The jack was about five feet high. You slipped it under the fender of a truck and it would lift the truck very easily. You could change a tire without having to get under the truck at all. It was a precision tool that cost well over a hundred dollars. Franklin reached for his fender-jack and unhooked it from his screen. He walked over to my truck and placed it in the back.

"That's a jack," he said. "You get caught with a flat in a snowstorm and you'll have that tire changed in a few seconds."

"Franklin, I can't take your jack. You need it—"

"I'll get another one. I want you to have it. I don't want you freezing to death in the snow. I want you to be alive when I come up there to visit."

We embraced. I suddenly realized how strange it would be not to see him anymore. "Thanks for the jack, Franklin," I said. "I'm going to miss you."

"I'll miss you too," Franklin said as he got into his truck. He turned on the ignition and paused for a moment before driving off. Leaning out the open window he added: "I'll see you in a year."

He drove down the road. I stood watching until I saw his truck pull up to his house and saw him go in. We both knew that his cancer might return any time. I wondered if I would ever see him again.

Moe's River

Dave's Nose

IT'S FIVE A.M. again in Moe's River. The woodstove's started. It's snowing gently. The coffee's perked. I'll fill you in on what happened after we left San Pedro. During our last few weeks there, I found an ad in a Canadian medical journal placed by a doctor in a small town in Quebec who wanted a partner. I wrote and said I was interested.

We arrived in the town to discover the doctor hadn't mentioned that it surrounded a pulp and paper mill, and the town and the countryside for miles around smelled like a sulphur pit. I agreed to work with him in the town but began to look for somewhere else to live. We returned to our truck and drove until the smell was gone. That brought us to Moe's River which was twenty miles away. Since we had just driven from New Mexico to Quebec, twenty miles didn't seem very far. In Moe's River we found a farm for rent on a mountaintop overlooking a valley.

Right from the beginning, on arriving home from work I would find sick people from Moe's River knocking on our door. These four or five people I would see in the evening upstairs in an extra bedroom were more of a strain for me than the twenty-five or thirty people I'd seen during the day. After a few months, I borrowed money from the bank and bought the farm we had been renting and had an office built in the attic. I'm now sitting writing and watching the snow fall at that office window.

The main reason we'd moved from San Pedro was because schooling didn't seem feasible there. The school in Moe's River was excellent; the teachers were competent and dedicated. There were only seventy-two students in the school: everyone knew everybody. The children in grade seven had to help the younger childen take off and put on their snowsuits in the winter. The grade seven school play was the most important annual event in Moe's River.

The school was a Protestant school where old-time country religion prevailed. Mark and Allen were the only Jews who ever attended it. At times they were referred to in the Old Testament term of "Hebrews"—as if they had wandered out of the Sinai desert to register in Moe's River Elementary School. From the moment they began attending, the school curriculum was modified to include teaching about the Jewish religion. It was a variant of the outlaw status I had been accorded in Fort Collins.

Since our farm was five miles out of town, the school bus picked up the boys in the morning and brought them home in the afternoon. Every morning, the boys and I, and Bingo, our one hundred and seventy-pound Newfoundland, would wait at the roadside for the school bus. We waited in autumn, often hearing honking overhead and looking up to see geese flying south in their relentless "V" formation. We waited through winter beside a snow Great Wall of China left taller each night by the snowblower—and which by midwinter was twice the height of the bus. We waited through early summer as Bingo lurched half-heartedly after butterflies. Whatever season it was, to the delight of all the kids on the bus, Bingo would always chase the bus for about a hundred yards or so, until it pulled away from him and rounded a corner that took it out of sight. When it was gone it would make me think of what it would be like someday when the boys would be older and be leaving home. What would Bingo and I do in the morning if there was no school bus to wait for? There's an old radiologist at the hospital in Sherbrooke, who I see once a week when I review the X-rays of patients I've sent in from Moe's River. He was once talking about his children who had long ago left home and were now living in other cities: "It's like a dream that's over—something beautiful that almost didn't happen—because it all went by so quickly."

A few months later, the radiologist, who was the only radiologist in the hospital, developed a cough which persisted for a few weeks. He ordered an X-ray of his own chest and took the film into his office to read it. He put it on the viewing screen on which he had read thousands of other people's X-rays over the years, and found himself staring at a chest in which there was a massive tumour in one lung, and a moderately-sized tumour in the other. He was dead within three months, and knew he would be from his first glance at his films. A few weeks after he had seen the films he said to me: "Do you remember what I said to you a few months ago, about it all being like a dream, when we were talking about children and their leaving? It's true of the whole process, I mean your own life—it's like a very brief dream that almost didn't happen."

We came to know most of the people in Moe's River very quickly.

People we didn't meet through my practice, or through the boys at school, I would come to know when Bingo went wandering — which he did frequently — and I had to find him. I met a good number of the townspeople one Saturday morning when he ended up in the basement of Moe's River Hotel and nobody could coax him out of it. Bingo was as stubborn as he was enormous. Four men pushing together were unable to force him up the stairs. They had even placed a large steak at the top of the stairs but it hadn't influenced him at all.

"He's afraid of stairs," I explained, after sheepishly apologizing for his being there in the first place.

"Let's set up the ramp we use for loading beer," said one of the barkeeper's assistants.

A panel was removed from one of the walls at ground level, and a ramp was placed leading up to the opening. Immediately, on his own, without needing one word of encouragement, Bingo ran up the ramp to the outside. He had wanted to get out the whole time. He's very shy. I'm sure he hated being the center of all this attention.

Another of Bingo's fears was thunder and lightning. Whenever we had a storm with thunder and lightning, he would immediately leap up and tear out of our house and head for a little cabin down the road where a friend of ours lived. She was a single mother who had built a cabin in the woods for herself and her daughter. It was so frail that Bingo could always push himself in the door. She could lock the door, but Bingo was so big and the door so flimsy, that she was afraid he would break it down. So she would let him in, dripping and panting, to take up most of the space in the cabin until the storm was over. For some reason he felt that frail shack was more secure against thunder and lightening than our solid, rambling farmhouse. We could never figure it out. When the storm was over, he would leave the cabin and slowly plod back up to our house at his usual elephantine pace.

If Bingo sounds dim-witted it's deceptive. He was probably very bright. This was clear in watching him play a quiet game of his design that occurred whenever the boys played catch. He would lie down near them and wait until they forgot about him. When one of them dropped the ball, or threw wildly, he would lunge for the ball, and would never miss getting it away from them. He would then swallow the ball to a point where they would have to reach elbow deep into his cavernous mouth to get it. Then he would lie down and wait until they forgot about him again, and repeat the whole sequence. He didn't want the ball. He just wanted to show them he was on top of the situation.

We also met people through the boys and their school friends. Mark had been the first to go to school. The first few weeks were difficult. Most of the children were from farming families. They had a vocabulary and a frame of reference that was different than the city life he had known originally, and life on the two Indian reservations he had known. Lenore happened to drive by the school one day at recess and saw him running by himself in a circle in the yard while the children played in groups. That picture haunted us. But within a few weeks he had a close and loyal friend. He was a boy named Pete Winston who came from a farming family with eight children. They lived about ten miles from us. When Mark visited there he would often stay for the weekend or for several days over holidays. Pete would sometimes stay over at our house, but only rarely and briefly, because he was needed at home for chores. A dairy farm is a living factory which requires fastidious and continuous attention. All of the Winston children woke at five in the morning to work in the stable. Towards breakfast-time the girls would leave the stable and help their mother prepare breakfast. In the evening there was more work in the stable. After school and on weekends there was work to be done in the garden, the fences, and in the chicken house. In spring the maple trees had to be tapped for maple syrup, and in summer hay had to be cut. For leisure, the boys and their father entered plowing and horse-pulling contests together; the girls and their mother entered cooking contests. When Mark stayed at the Winstons he worked with Pete at whatever Pete's chores were at a given moment. Through his visits to the Winstons he came to understand the lives his schoolmates were living, and through Mark and Pete's friendship a close and loyal relationship grew between our two families. I became their doctor, and they were always ready to help us with rural living.

Dave is a thirty-five year old alcoholic who used to be a personnel manager in a local factory but hasn't worked for several years. He's on welfare and lives in a tiny room in Moe's River Hotel. For an hour or two a day he helps the bartender load the bar with beer. This helps him pay for his drinking. It was Dave who had suggested using the ramp that time Bingo had wandered in to the basement of the hotel. Dave's face is completely disfigured by a huge, red, twisted drinker's nose.

On Dave's first visit to my office he cast a glance at a cup of coffee I had beside me on my desk and said:

"Coffee addict, eh?"

"Keeps me going," I answered. "Would you like some?"

"No thanks," Dave answered with a grin. "I have other vices."

"What brings you here today, Dave?" I asked. "What's the problem?"

I knew the problem. He had told my secretary, Lorraine, who has lived here all her life, and has known Dave since childhood, that someone had said I might be able to help him with his nose. I already knew what he was going to ask me. Here I was, asking "What's the problem?" when he was facing me with a nose that looked like a red, fleshy, and misshappen ball. It looked like someone had twisted it off the end of his face, stamped on it several times, and stuck it back on. It was as prominent between us as the bowl of porridge stuck on the nose of a husband in a fairy story about the poor old couple who had been granted three wishes:

Husband: "I wish for a big bowl of porridge."

Wife: "What a stupid thing to wish for! I wish that bowl of porridge was stuck on your nose!"

Of course they had to use the third wish to get the bowl of porridge off his nose. They were left as the same poor old couple. Except that now they were really mad at each other. Anyway, back to Dave and his nose:

"What's the problem, Dave?"

Even though I knew what he was here for I had no choice but to pretend I didn't. After all, I couldn't say: "Are you here about your nose?" or: "My secretary said you wanted to see me about your nose." It was like having Cyrano de Bergerac as a patient. I couldn't mention his nose unless he did.

"It's about my nose," Dave answered abjectly.

Good. That's over with. Now we could get on with it: "What about it?" I asked.

"It's red and swollen."

"How long has it been like that?"

"About five years. It began about two years after I started drinking heavily. But it's getting worse all the time."

"Did you ever see a doctor about it?" I asked.

"Once," Dave answered. "He said he couldn't do anything for it. Some of the guys at the hotel said they thought you could. Also now it seems infected. That's new."

The diagnosis: Rhinophyma. A nose like a rhinoceros. Drinker's nose. It can happen without drinking, but it's much more common in drinkers. I took out a dermatology book and looked up Rhinophyma. I showed Dave a picture of someone else with it. It was reassuring for Dave to know that his big, red nose was a known and classified entity — and someone else had one.

"Can you do something about it?" Dave asked.

"You can," I answered.

"I can't," he said.

"Have you ever gone to A.A....?"

"I guess I'll just have to live with a big red nose."

"It's an offer you can't afford to refuse. There's no A.A. in Moe's River. You'd have to go into Sherbrooke. At least three times a week."

Dave sat silently thinking for a moment. He looked out on the valley below us, and turned back to me and said in a tone that lacked his usual flippancy: "All right, I'll go."

"Good," I said. "Now let me ask you a few other things, and then we'll get back to your nose."

A few more questions revealed that Dave's nose was not his major problem. It was only a visible exclamation mark to a generally advanced state of alcoholic deterioration. He had pain in his belly and blood in his stools. He had no appetite, bruised easily and had periods of confusion. After more than a day of trying to stop drinking he would get the shakes. On physicial examination he had many signs of advanced liver disease: a hard liver, an enlarged spleen, enlarged breasts, dilated veins on his chest, and a roughening and reddening of his palms.

Eventually, cirrhosis ensues and the liver becomes a fibrous lump obstructing the flow of blood. This leads to internal bleeding. The liver normally removes ammonia gas, one of the waste products of metabolism, from the body. In liver failure ammonia gas accummulates in the brain and causes confusion. The liver also plays a role in blood clotting. It was clear why Dave was becoming confused, bleeding from his bowel, and bruising easily.

"Dave, you've got signs and symptoms of serious liver disease. If you don't stop drinking, you're going to die pretty soon. I want you to go into the hospital. The pain in your belly, the blood in you stool—"

"I figured you'd say that. When do you want me to go?"

"Today."

"All right."

Dave's resignation reminded me of an alcoholic I'd seen in an emergency room in my internship who had observed: "I was walking along the street and the world stopped," he'd said, and then added after a moment's reflection, "and I can't get it started again."

Dave went into the hospital in Sherbrooke that day. Sherbrooke is about thirty miles from Moe's River. Because of my workload in Moe's River, five days went by and it turned out impossible for me to get into see him. I had been getting reports from the doctors by telephone. Tests confirmed he had advanced cirrhosis. On admission he had symptoms of alcohol withdrawal, but delerium tremens had been avoided by giving him heavy doses of tranquilizers that he was now weaned from. Knowing I wouldn't be able to get into see him for a few more days, I phoned the nursing station on his ward and told the nurses to put him on the line.

Dave said he was feeling better than he'd felt in years. As far as his nose was concerned, at least the secondary infection was clearing. He thanked me for phoning and said he understood my not being able to get by. He spoke in a straightforward manner with none of his old flippancy. I could hear flashes of the former personnel manager in his voice: "Thanks Doc, I'm starting to feel like a person again."

Talking to Dave on the phone reminded me of the time in internship when I was at a patient's bedside as she began to wake from a suicide attempt. What do you say to someone waking into a world after they've tried to kill themselves? I'd seen a psychiatrist handle that moment by waiting ten minutes till the patient spoke first. That's enough to make anyone want to try again immediately. I watched this woman stir and wondered what I was going to say. She was a tiny woman of about thirty-five who had overdosed on a massive number of sleeping pills, and had been brought in comatose. Judging from the number of pills she had taken there was no questionning the validity of her attempt. It had not been a gesture. During the night she had been on a respirator and her stomach had been pumped. Litres of fluid had been poured into her veins to flush out the drug. Her stirrings progressed into movements, and suddenly she opened her eyes, and they fell on me: "Are you glad you're alive?" I asked.

"I don't know," she answered.

"I am," I said.

She reached out and took my hand and said: "That's the first kind thing anyone's said to me in thirty years."

Dave didn't drink for three weeks after discharge from the hospital. He went to A.A. meetings three times a week. Everyone at Moe's River Hotel was amazed at his abstinence, and the improved appearance of his nose. On the Sunday of the third week he got drunk. He came by that afternoon with a friend who was having chest pain. The friend, a middle-aged man named Bobby, was also one of the town's heavier drinkers. Unlike Dave he had a family and a job, but usually spent a good part of the weekend drinking with Dave in Moe's River Hotel. He had just eaten Sunday dinner with his family. His chest pain was probably indigestion, but it was worrying him and preventing him from drinking. I explained to him that it was probably indigestion, but that I would do an electrocardiagram to make sure it wasn't a heart attack. Allen and I had been playing catch outside when they came. Bingo had succeeded in swallowing our ball three times in twenty minutes. When Bobby came with the chest pain, I asked Allen if he wanted to help me do an electrocardiagram. He was six years old at the time, and like Mark who was eight, he was interested in my work. I would take them on house calls. I also taught them about how the different systems in the body work. I knew he'd enjoy doing the electrocardiagram, and it was also a way I could go on having some time with him even though I'd be working.

"The heart's a muscle," I explained to Bobby, as I showed Allen how to attach the electrodes to his arms and legs. "A kind of electrical force goes through the heart as it contracts. That's what we're measuring. If the heart is in some kind of trouble, we'll see it in the pattern this pen is tracing on the paper as I move this electrode over your chest."

Despite the fact Bobby wasn't listening, and just wanted to know he wasn't having a heart attack and could go drinking, and Dave was pretending to listen but was too drunk to concentrate, I couldn't stop explaining what I was doing. It's a kind of habit I've gotten into. Most people do appreciate knowing what you're doing to them, and why you're doing it, but Bobby couldn't have cared less.

The electrocardiogram was normal. Bobby left with some antacid. Allen and I went back to playing catch and prying the ball out of Bingo's cavernous mouth. About an hour later I was upstairs in my office, and I heard Allen talking to Lenore in the kitchen:

"The heart's a muscle," he was telling her. "It runs on its own kind of electricity that you can actually measure with the electrocardiagram machine. Dad taught me how to—"

The phone's ringing. Anyway, you get the idea. Bobby didn't care about the heart being a muscle. But Allen did. The phone call is from a schoolteacher from a nearby village, who had been up early chopping firewood, and cut his finger.

"Don't ring the bell," I tell him. "the family's still sleeping. I'm up. I'll hear you on the stairway."

I like sewing up cuts. There's something refreshingly finite about the process. Confronted with so many unknowns, and so many insoluble illnesses, I find something satisfying in sewing together two edges of a jagged wound. It's easier than trying to help someone like Dave.

I had two other phone calls during the night. One was at eleven-thirty. It was from one of our neighbours calling about her brother who lived five miles away in another town. I saw him about a back problem about two months ago. He's a logger who has had back pain off and on for several years. It was a chronic strain that probably could have been cured by physiotherapy and corrective exercises in the long run, but for the moment I had given him an anti-inflammatory pill which reduces the swelling and pain. I mentioned the physiotherapy and corrective exercises, but I knew he would never do them. I knew for him there was something emasculating about that kind of treatment. He would have been happier if I said he should have surgery. That would have given his symptom the kind of status and masculinity he felt was appropriate. He had returned after a week on the pills. They were wonderful. His pain was gone. But there was one problem: "They took away the back pain," he said, "but they left me unable to raise," he added, pointing to his penis.

I knew it was most likely not so. There are pills which can cause impotence as a side-effect — but not anti-inflammatory pills. They're just glorified aspirins. Like aspirins they can cause fatal bleeding ulcers. But they don't cause impotence. If he had a disc problem in his back, and it were severe enough, it could cause impotence as a result of spinal nerve compression, but X-rays of his back had not suggested a disc injury. The waiting room was crowded. I had thought this follow-up visit for a back problem was going to need about ten minutes. Now I was faced with a full-scale enquiry into all the complex conditions which could lead to impotence — such as diabetes and multiple sclerosis. I did a detailed neurological examination to make sure there were no other deficits in his nervous system. Only after forty minutes of this had gone by, did it occur to me to ask about the extent of his problem:

"How long has this been going on for?" I asked.

"I don't have it any more," he answered. "it only happened one night. I stopped the pill for a day, and the next day it was O.K.. I'm back on the pills now and there's no problem."

That visit was about a month ago. I'd figured as I usually do, that no news was good news. When his sister called at eleven-thirty last night, I didn't imagine the news would be good: "What's the problem?" I asked.

"My brother's house burned down tonight!"

"My God! That's terrible! Is anyone hurt?"

"No."

I couldn't understand why she was phoning me at eleven-thirty at night if nobody was hurt, but nevertheless I said: "I'm sorry to hear about the fire. Is there anything I can do?"

"The pills," she said in a desolate voice, "— the ones you gave him for his back, — they were lost in the fire."

"Don't worry. I have lots more."

"Good, I'll be there first thing in the morning."

I didn't ask her why she was calling me at eleven-thirty. In the midst of this bad luck they were clinging to a good thing that had happened lately. Her brother had found a pill that takes away his back pain. If he took the physiotherapy and did the exercises he wouldn't need the pill. But therapeutic exercises didn't fit in his cosmology. If the ailment he'd been complaining of all these years could be cured by exercises, it would be robbed of all its stature. He needed to give it the mystique of an illness like diabetes where pills or injections were needed daily. It was his way of cutting off the moose's head before dragging it through the camp.

The second call I had during the night was just after midnight. It was from an elderly lady with a quavering voice: "I'm Mrs. Abigail Johnston. You don't know me. But I'm a neighbour of Ethel Sparks."

I didn't know Ethel Sparks either.

"Of whom?" I said sleepily. Getting up in the middle of the night to answer the phone is not something that gets easier each time, or that you can train for like an athlete trains at a sport and increases his endurance at it. It's always newly and totally unendurable.

"Ethel Sparks," the old lady's quavering voice continued in an admonishing tone for my not remembering. "You saw her once about two years ago. She lives midway between Scotstown and Milan. Her husband used to own the general store in Middlebury until he became too ill to manage it. Then he died, of course, and—"

Mrs. Johnston would have gone all night recounting the life and times of Ethel Sparks, but now that I was waking up, I did remember seeing the lady once two years ago.

"I remember," I interrupted. "She had severe anemia from a bleeding ulcer. I had her put in the hospital under Dr. Morrison —"

"That's right," said Mrs. Johnston. "They gave her blood and then sent her to a convalescent home. But she didn't like it there at all and discharged herself against Dr. Morrison's advice and—"

"But what's happening tonight — now — at twelve-thirty?" I interrupted.

"That's just what I was trying to tell you when you interrupted," she countered testily. "She didn't like the nursing home and her son took her out—"

"That's two years ago. What's happening TONIGHT? NOW? AT TWELVE-THIRTY?"

"Well, that's what I'm trying to tell you. But you keep interrupting. For the last two years she has been living at home with her son. A few months ago her son met a girl from Montreal. About a week ago he decided to go live with that girl in Montreal. Some people say she's pregnant. I wouldn't know but—"

"Mrs. Johnston, so far I don't see what this has to do with me. Just tell me, what's the problem that led you to call me tonight at—"

"What's the problem?" she said with incredulous exasperation. "You're a doctor and you don't see the problem? You think it's right for a son to leave a sick old woman like that alone?"

"Look, Mrs. Johnston, I'm sure you're right. It sounds like it would be better if she weren't living alone. But why are you phoning me tonight after midnight?"

"Because I just found out about it," she answered.

"Mrs. Johnston, this is something that involves Mrs. Sparks and her son and her family and friends. The way I see it, it doesn't really involve me, but I'll speak to you tomorrow about it. Right now I'm too tired to talk any more about it."

"You'll call me tomorrow for sure?" she asked.

"Yes," I said, not quite believing that this was really ending.

"First thing?" she said.

"Maybe not first thing," I said. "But tomorrow for sure."

"In the morning?"

I was losing strength. I wanted to explain if there were other more urgent problems demanding attention, I would attend to them first — but sleep was beckoning, and I capitulated and muttered begrudgingly:

"In the morning."

When I had gotten up at four forty-five this morning, I thought of calling back Mrs. Johnston. The conversation would have gone something like this: "Hello, Mrs. Johnston?"

"Yes, this is Mrs. Johnston," a sleepy, old, puzzled, quavering voice would answer.

"I know how to solve Ethel Spark's problem."

"Oh, yes?" she would say, shaking herself from sleep.

"Yes. She can move in with you," I would say brightly.

"Yes, I suppose she could," she would answer reluctantly and then probably would add, "But what time is it? It's still dark out!"

"It's four forty-five," I would say cheerfully.

"Doctor, it's an interesting idea you have there about Ethel moving in with us, but why are you calling me so early in the morning to tell me about it?"

"Because I just thought of it," I would answer.

I hear Réjean moving about downstairs in our kitchen. He's probably attaching a hose to our kitchen sink to run some water to the barn. He has to do that when the pipes in the barn freeze—which they do from time to time. The cattle in the barn are getting angry at the delay. I can hear them bellowing. I go down to the kitchen to say hello: "You have it tough, Réjean," I tell him. "Up from five in the morning 'till eleven at night, repairing one broken thing after another."

"I know someone else who gets up at five." Réjean answered.

"But I don't have to deal with broken things all day. That would be a nightmare for me."

"But I don't have to deal with the public. That would be a nightmare for me," Réjean responded as he tightened the hose onto the faucet. "But speaking of something not working the way it should, my dad has been having a strange problem the last few days. Whenever he starts to speak he breaks into tears. We thought it was just something strange that would go away, but it hasn't. I'd appreciate it if you could get a look at him today—"

"I will for sure. That is really strange."

"Do you have any idea what it could be?"

"It could be some kind of stroke—a short circuit caused by a loss of circulation in some area of the brain. I'd like to think of something else. For the moment I can't." I thought of a brain tumour but didn't mention it. "I'll see him first thing today. I'll go over there before the office starts."

"It looks like your office is starting already," Réjean said. "There's a guy coming up the stairs."

"It's a schoolteacher from St. Malo who cut his hand chopping wood," I said as I went to intercept the patient on the stairs—in case he forgot and rang the bell.

I tried to hoard as much satisfaction as I could in sewing up the school teacher's finger. I knew I would need it when facing how little I could probably do for Réjean's father, and how little I had done for Dave.

Meet me at the Crossroads

IT WAS ONE A.M. and a snowstorm that had been starting up when I had gone to bed at eleven had gathered momentum. It was a thick storm with soft heavy flakes winding in at the windshield from somewhere out where—my younger son Allen, now eight-years-old says —there is no end: "Space has no end," he muses to himself. "It goes on forever," he would add.

I had been wakened up at 12:45 by a phone call about Lisa Macdowell, a ten year old girl who was having abdominal pain and vomiting. The Macdowells lived about ten miles away. I knew approximately where they lived but wasn't quite sure: "Meet me at the crossroads," I'd told them, "and I'll follow you from there."

Now that the shock of waking from sleep was over and the overwhelming desire just to crawl back to bed had passed, I was enjoying the peace of the storm. There was no phone in the truck. There was nothing to do but drive along and watch the heavy snowflakes hit the windshield.

As I was starting to wonder if I'd gotten lost, I saw lights up ahead. A pick-up truck was parked at the crossroads. The lights flashed as I approached. The truck began moving and I followed behind it. We moved slowly along in the storm for several miles until we reached a farm where the truck pulled in.

When I entered the farmhouse, the father and three of his sons were sitting at the kitchen table. The son who had driven to the crossroads to meet me sat down beside them. The four sons were all in their twenties. Lisa, the ten year old girl whom I'd been called to see, was born at least ten years after the youngest of the sons, and was doted on by the whole family. Even though the four sons would all be getting up at five in the morning to milk the cows, they were all sitting up waiting to see what I would say about Lisa.

The mother was in Lisa's room. I examined Lisa and felt relatively safe that she had a flu rather than an appendicitis:

"I think it's a flu," I said to Mrs. Macdowell. "But we have to keep appendicitis in mind. I can give her something for the nausea, but I can't give her anything for pain. We have to see what becomes of it. Hopefully it will pass off within a few hours. On the other hand, if it gets worse or moves down to her lower right side, let me know right away. I'll call you in the morning to see how she's doing."

I made a summary for the men in the kitchen — a wave of relief flashed over their faces.

I drove home hoping I wouldn't miss the crossroads. The storm was growing thicker. I wished it would go on for days.

Two Bad Guys

I WAS EXPECTING LORRAINE, my secretary, to send in the next patient when she came in and said: "There's two police officers who want to see you. Should I send them in before the next patient?"

"I guess so. I wonder who it's about."

Two lean and muscled men in their thirties entered the office. They looked very sure of themselves. "Doctor, I'm constable Fortin and this is constable Emmet. We're from the Royal Canadian Mounted Police. We have some questions we'd like to ask you."

"Have a seat," I said, gesturing to the chairs in front of my desk. I wondered which patient it was about.

They flashed their I.D. cards as they sat down. They looked even more sure of themselves in their photos. They put their identity cards away and the spokesman produced a small photo of a young black man and placed it on my desk in front of me. It was Bill.

"Do you recognize this man?" the spokesman asked.

"No," I answered.

My "no" sounded very hollow. Even to me. It sounded as if it were coming from underwater. I felt as if I were watching one of those crime shows on T.V. that I see my kids watching as I pass the living room. Except now I was in it, and not on the right side. And everyone knows the mounties always get their man.

"You signed a passport application for him five years ago," the spokesman continued self-assuredly. "As you know, when you sign a passport you confirm that you have known this person for two years prior to signing the application."

"I don't know him. And I don't remember signing his passport," I answered from underwater.

"Doctor," the spokesman said solemnly, "I think you should know before we go any further that the penalty for endorsing a fraudulent passport application can be two years in prison."

"There's something else you should know," the second officer added, speaking for the first time: "The man in the photo was arrested in Copenhagen a week ago. He's being held as a suspect in a case we're not at will to discuss at this moment. At the time of his arrest he was carrying a fraudulent Canadian passport for which you were the guarantor."

"Somebody must have forged my signature," I countered lamely.

"We have copies of your signature from your driver's license application and your income tax return. It matches the one on the passport."

"So what if it matches? That could just mean that it was good forgery," I answered.

Their smug self-assuredness was irritating. The mounties may always get their man, but I was going to make them work for it. "Doctor," said the second constable, "we don't think it was a forgery. We think you signed the application."

He paused and looked straight into my eyes. He was hoping that I would break down and admit he was right. Their behaviour worried me. Everyone knows that when there are two cops one acts as the bad guy, and the other as the good. Here the second officer who was now beginning to speak was more menacing than the first. It didn't auger well. I wondered what Bill had done in Copenhagen.

"But just to give you the benefit of the doubt," the second officer continued when he saw his pause was non-productive, "we're going to submit the signature to a computerized handwriting analyzer we have in Ottawa. If it says, as we think it will, that it's your signature, we'll be back. If it says it isn't your signature, we'll drop the whole issue. In order to do this we need you to sign your name ten times on a piece of paper, and give it to us to put into the machine along with the passport application."

For the first time since they had shown me Bill's photo I felt a small surge of hope — about as much as a boxer might feel lying flat on his back half unconscious with the referee hovering over him counting:

"Seven...eight...nine..."

One of my eyes was closed from a cut over my lid; blood from a gash in my lip was streaming down my chin. But there was hope! If the computerized handwriting analysis machine was anywhere near as unreliable as some of our medical machines, there was probably a five to ten percent chance that I might get a false exoneration. I staggered up from the floor of the ring and wrote my name ten times — trying as much as possible to subtly infuse some variation into my signature.

The officers took the paper with the ten signatures and rose to leave. "We'll be back," said the one who had become the new spokesman.

Two bad guys. It didn't look good.

Bill was a patient I had treated many years earlier for a kidney infection when I was working as a resident in the emergency room of one of the hospitals. I had received a phone call at home from someone who was kind of an acquaintance rather than a friend. He could be classified as a friend of a friend. His name was Philippe. He was a sculptor.

"I need your help," Philippe said.

"What is it?" I asked warily. I had just worked a twenty-four hour shift. The phone call woke me up.

"I've got a very sick man I'd like you to see."

"What's the problem?"

"He's probably got a kidney infection. He has a defect in his kidneys that he was born with and apparently it's very dangerous for him to have an infection."

"O.K., I can help you out. I can't do it myself at this moment. I just worked twenty-four hours and I'm sleeping. I'm on again at the hospital at six tonight. He could see me there then. If he's so sick that he needs to be seen right away you'd better take him to the emergency right now."

"He can't go to the hospital," Philippe said.

"Why not?" I answered, starting to get irritated.

"He's a political fugitive," Philippe answered.

"What do you mean?" I asked with increasing irritation.

This was getting to be a lengthy conversation. I wanted to get back to sleep. I had worked every moment of the previous twenty-four hours and was desperately tired. "He's a Black Panther. He's here illegally. He jumped bail on a trumped-up charge for sedition. The only thing he's ever done is to try and organize black people to fight for their rights. If he goes to a hospital, he could be arrested. He's trying to get to Europe or Cuba as quick as possible. But now he's sick."

"O.K., bring him by here to my house at five just before I go to the hospital. I'll be up and recovered by then. Tell him to bring a urine sample in a bottle. Sterilize the bottle by boiling it in water and allowing it to cool. I can bring the urine to the hospital for culture to identify the microbe."

Bill was sick. He had a fever of 103. There's a bedside diagnostic sign for kidney infection. You tap the patient in the angle between the ribs and the vertebral column. If it's unduly painful he probably has infection in that kidney. When I tapped him, Bill jumped and howled in pain. I had my diagnosis. On a return visit three days later Bill was essentially well. He accepted the kidney punch with equanimity. The culture was growing a microbe that was susceptible to the antibiotic I had placed him on. I told him to stay on the antibiotic another week and come back with a urine sample for retesting. Philippe, the sculptor, had come with him on these visits. On the last visit Philippe said: "We appreciate the help you've given Bill, but there's something else we'd like to ask you. You know why he's here. You understand he's got to get to Europe. The FBI and the CIA are after him. We need you to sign a passport application for him. It says it can be a doctor or a lawyer or a minister. Obviously he's not a Canadian, and the whole thing is a falsification, but we've been assured that with a legitimate endorser like yourself that it will work."

"Look, Philippe, I'm sympathetic to what Bill's working for, but if I'm caught doing this I'll lose my license, and that would be the end of my work."

"I understand Doc," Bill said. "I don't want you to do anything that you really don't feel you should."

I signed the application.

The two RCMP officers had visited me on a Friday afternoon. The next morning, a sunny Saturday morning, I drove into town to buy a weekend paper and passed the same two officers driving the opposite direction toward our farm. I pretended I didn't notice them even though I passed within a few feet of their car. When I picked up a paper at the grocery store there was a headline about the discovery of an AIM or American Indian Movement "underground railway" between Indian reservations in New Mexico and Arizona and reservations in the Northwest Territories. It described how AIM members were obtaining false passports and weapons. It mentioned two reservations I had worked on.

I had once treated some AIM militants who were hiding out in Fort Collins. I guessed the RCMP was working me up as some kind of international agent of sedition in medical clothing. I expected to find them at the farm when I returned, and was greatly relieved to find they weren't there. I figured they just wanted to get a look at it from the car. Maybe they thought they would spot a cache of weapons through a barn window, or find a helioport disguised as a haystack.

I didn't hear anything from them for nine months. I thought maybe the handwriting machine had really fouled up like I'd hoped it would. Or I thought maybe they had found I wasn't part of an international ring of sedition, and had simply signed one passport. I say maybe because deep down I thought they'd be back. The mounties always get their man,

One day when I was working at the emergency room at the hospital, the receptionist who registers patients outside in the waiting room approached me and said: "Doctor, there's three officers out in the waiting room who say they would like to speak to you."

I asked another doctor to cover the emergency room for me and took the three officers into an empty room. There were the two who

I already knew and an older man, probably a senior officer brought along to crack my resistance. The new man spoke first. There was a profound weariness to his voice. It implied he'd dealt with countless liars like me and always won in the end: "The handwriting analysis machine says it's your signature. There's no possibility of forgery. The machine has never been wrong."

He paused and let this news sink in. He took out Bill's photo and placed it on a desk in front of me and continued: "Doctor," he said with great weariness, "you did sign that passport application, didn't you?"

"I don't care what the machine says," I answered with weariness to equal his. "Somebody forged my name."

"Doctor," he sighed with even more weariness and some disgust, "we've come all the way from Ottawa to give you one last chance to tell the truth. If you do we can probably get you off completely. We just want to know why you did it, so we can better understand how these kinds of breakdowns in the system occur. That's all. We wouldn't have to prosecute you."

I had to admit this older guy was good. Part of me really wanted to end the whole thing and let him take care of me. But the thought of being at his mercy held me back. Instead I found myself answering: "These visits are wasting a lot of my time. I have to get back to the emergency room. All I can tell you is I didn't sign that man's passport application. I've got to get back to work."

"O.K. Doc, have it your way," said the older man. "This is your turf. We'll leave now. But we'll see you again on ours. Soon. And then it'll be too late to make any deals. You just blew your last chance. Go out and take care of those people in the emergency room. They'll be among the last people you'll ever treat."

That night I phoned a lawyer who I knew. "You're crazy!" he said. "I'll phone them and tell them you'll talk."

Three weeks went by and I heard nothing from the lawyer. I phoned him and asked:

"What did they say?"

"What do you mean what did they say?" the lawyer asked. "I told you to phone them and say you'd talk," he said.

"I thought you said you would phone them." I answered.

He phoned them the next day and called me back to report: "It's too late. Now they're not interested. They're out to get you."

A few days later two RCMP officers delivered a summons for me to appear in court in a month. The lawyer tried again to tell them I would talk. They weren't interested.

On the day of the court hearing, the crown lawyer let my lawyer know he was willing to make a deal. If I plead guilty he would ask for leniency.

I pleaded guilty. My lawyer pointed out to the judge that I had taken no money for signing the passport. He argued that I was a doctor serving society in isolated areas, and that I should not be penalized harshly for this one offence. I was convicted but given a suspended sentence. There would be no penalty as long as I was not involved in any further passport irregularities.

Lenore met Philippe in Montreal several weeks later. In the intervening years Philippe had won several government awards and commissions for his sculpture. He no longer dabbled in radical politics. "I understand your husband was visited by the RCMP about that passport he signed for that Black Panther," Philippe said to Lenore.

"How did you know?" Lenore asked him.

Philippe ignored her question.

"I hope he didn't mention my name," he said.

Or a Doctor

LYELL EVANS was a forty-nine year old man who died a year ago in heart surgery in an operation I had advised him to have. His death had been the result of a mechanical failure in an oxygenating machine. A second machine brought in to replace the first one was also defective. At the time of his death, Lyell's wife, Monica, was going to accept the hospital's apologies and let the matter end there. I told her that machines being defective were somebody's fault, and apologies weren't going to help her support her four children. She saw a lawyer. The oxygenating machine company is going to have to pay compensation. But nobody is going to replace Lyell.

Lyell had worked in the papermill in the sulphur smelling town I had first worked in before I had set up office in Moe's River. One night while bowling he had a massive heart attack. He survived but was left with chest pain that proved to be medically unmanageable. There was no choice but to do a coronary artery by-pass operation. A successful operation could render him pain-free. There was a one or two percent chance of not surviving the operation. It took Lyell less than five seconds to make his decision. He wanted to be a normal husband and father again.

When the machines failed, Lyell was left without oxygen to his brain for nine minutes. After the operation he was kept alive for three days but repeated electroencephalographic recordings showed no evidence of electrical activity. He could be kept alive on machines for an indefinite period, but he would never be a person again. On the fourth day, Lyell was declared brain dead. I had gone with Monica to see him several times over those three days. He was surrounded by a hopeless litany of thudding respirators, sucking drains and beeping monitors. After all the plugs were pulled, and all the mechanical bluffing was over, he died within a minute. It was frightening how quickly Lyell looked dead; there is something very fragile inside each of us that a corpse doesn't have.

Monica was a nervous woman who had always leaned on Lyell for support. The four children ranged in age from eleven to sixteen. They were used to relying on Lyell for support as well. Since his death, Monica had been doing her best to be both parents, but everyone was finding it hard.

Yesterday Monica brought in Bruce, the twelve year old, because he was having headaches. He's been having headaches for several months and they'd gotten worse over the last few weeks. His examination was normal. "They're what are called tension headaches, Bruce," I explained. "When you're feeling tense or worried about something your scalp muscles tighten and it gives you a headache. Anybody who's gone through what you've gone through with your dad's death could get them easily enough."

Tears came to Bruce's eyes. I went over and sat beside him.

"I have a paper route," Bruce said, and began to cry softly. "There's this dumb ten-year-old kid who's always taking papers out of my sack when my back is turned. I caught him doing it one morning last week.

Just as I had grabbed him his mother put her head out the window. She wouldn't listen to anything about him taking papers. She said I was a bully and that anyone could see from the way I behaved that I had no father."

"That's terrible—"

"Doctor," Bruce sobbed, "why'd he die?"

"He died because those machines failed. It was an inexcusable mistake. He knew there was some danger in the operation, but what happened was out of nowhere."

"I remember him explaining before the operation that he was taking it so that he could be a normal father again." Bruce said. "He told us that the night before, and then we never heard him speak again."

"But you know what he would want for you. And you're doing it all: taking care of your mother, doing well in school, the paper route, —looking after things—just like he did—"

"Do you think my dad is watching me all the time?" Bruce asked.

"I'm sure he is," I said, "and he always will be. I know Lyell. He wouldn't miss your growing up for anything. He'll be watching it all. Do you have any idea what you want to do when you're older?"

"I want to be a stuntman or a doctor," Bruce answered.

I really laughed. Most people might see a paradox there. I didn't. He had managed to state precisely what I'd always felt about my work— that I was on a tightrope over a canyon of uncertainty, with only a few tired facts and a lot of theories for a balancing pole.

"You'll be great at either, Bruce," I said.

The stunt for the moment was helping him with his headaches. I called in his mother and explained his headaches were from tension, and told her to give him some Aspirin when they persisted, and that I wanted to see him every few weeks for a while to see what we could do about reducing the tension he was feeling. There was a painful sense of Lyell's profound absence hovering over us.

We are all stuntmen.

As Good as Dead

IT WAS A CLEAR AUTUMN MORNING. For a few years now I've been running several miles a day. On my run early this morning, I passed the house of a patient named Eugene Desrosiers, whom I had put in the hospital the day before.

When I'd seen Eugene yesterday he was extremely dehydrated; his eyes were sunken and his mouth was dry; his skin was loose and creased. I tested his urine and found it full of sugar. Eugene had never shown any signs of diabetes in the past, but now he was close to becoming comatose. After taking a blood sample to confirm the elevation of sugar in his blood, I began intravenous treatment with fluid and insulin, and called for an ambulance to take him the thirty miles to the hospital.

I had phoned late last night and early this morning to find out how Eugene was doing. Both reports were favourable. He was doing well. His blood sugar had returned to normal. Over the next few days it would be determined how much insulin he would need to keep it normal. He would be coming home in a few days. I thought I would stop in and give his wife this encouraging news.

I approached Eugene's house warily. They had a vicious-looking dog who would growl at me when I ran by or entered the house. Eugene or his wife would always call him off and he would be satisfied with glowering at me. As I cautiously drew near the door of the house, the dog suddenly appeared from around the corner. It was only then that I realized Eugene's wife was probably at the hospital with him. I should have realized there was no car outside the house. And there was no one home to control the dog. He snarled happily, bared his teeth, and prepared to lunge.

Suddenly the door of the house opened. A gnarled old man with skeletal fingers beckoned for the dog to desist. The dog growled and went slowly back around the corner from where he had come. You could sense his bitter disappointment in the reluctant pace at which he moved. It was as if he was hoping the old man would change his mind.

I had forgotten that Eugene's ninety-year old father lived with them. He had a room upstairs. I'd never met him before, I was very glad to meet him now. I had come bearing good news and I was determined to share it.

"Ca va mieux avec Eugène," I said to the old man.

(Eugene is doing better.)

"Qu'est-ce qu'il a?" the old man asked.

(What does he have?)

"Il fait du diabète. Mais c'est déjà controllé," I answered.

(He had diabetes. But it's already under control.)

"Diabète?" the old man questioned solemnly.

(Diabetes?)

"Oui," I answered. "Mais il va mieux—".

("Yes,") I answered. ("But he's doing well and—")

"Quasiment fini," the old man said and shut the door.

(As good as dead.)

I ran on home. It was mid-morning but the moon was still up over the yellow hayfields. It was the peak of autumn. In the surrounding hills, the red and orange leaves of the hardwood trees contrasted with the evergreens. Farmers were turning over the soil and plowing in fertilizer for winter. I was grateful when it was cow shit and ran faster when it was pig shit.

The old man had seen a lot of people die. And they all had doctors. And some of these people had probably died not long after a doctor had said they were doing better. But Eugene had gone out his door looking three-quarters dead and would return looking well. Quasiment guéri—(as good as cured.)

Three Days Late

I COULD TELL as I accepted the call that the long distance operator's accent was from somewhere in the American Southwest:

"Go ahead," the operator said.

"Doctor?" the caller queried.

"Yes," I answered.

"It's Franklin—"

"Franklin!"

"I'm calling from a phone booth in Idaho," Franklin said. "We're going to be about three days late."

"Late for what?" I asked.

"Don't you remember?" Franklin asked. "I told you that I would visit you in Canada a year after you left San Pedro. It's a year today."

I remembered Franklin saying he would visit in a year, but I had always thought of it as a kind of wish, rather than something he would ever really carry out. I was delighted he was coming. I was also relieved that he wasn't calling to tell me that the cancer of his stomach had recurred. That was the first thought I had when I heard his voice. "I knew you'd come, Franklin," I lied, "but I didn't realize a year had gone by. Things have gone so fast here."

Lenore and I were both eager to see Franklin again. I was also pleased that Mark and Allen would be able to make a connection with San Pedro again. Several months ago, when Mark and I were driving into Moe's River, we passed a young man in a pick-up truck who was wearing an old brown cowboy hat tipped over one eye.

"He looks like Clifford—the Apache guy who died in that car accident," Mark said. "Remember? He gambled with me with a Chanukah dredyl for a whole night just before he died?"

"Just what I was thinking," I answered.

"I hope there's someone else growing up like him in San Pedro." Mark said.

On another occasion, when we were talking about honesty being a rare quality in people Mark had said: "Franklin always told the truth."

Franklin arrived three days later in his pick-up truck with Mattie, a woman named Adele, and three of her children. One of the children was a niece Adele adopted when her sister died. Later Franklin told me how her sister died, and asked if I remembered the incident. I would never forget it. It goes back to that Sunday afternoon in San Pedro when I had been called to her house after her husband shot her and then killed himself. The adopted niece was one of the children I'd seen wandering around the house crying that afternoon.

Franklin did his best to make the visit work. Since we had a farm, he was determined we start keeping a few head of beef cattle. He went with us to a cattle auction to buy them, and taught us how to care for them. He helped Lenore with the chickens and weeded the garden. He cooked chili and tacos. But the visit was a disaster. It didn't work. Adele drank heavily and she beat her children. She never did it in front of us, but we could hear sounds of scuffle from behind a closed door, and one of the children would emerge crying or sulking a few minutes later.

"Franklin, either you stop her or I will," I told him.

"Don't you think I've tried," he answered. "She stops for a few days, then she gets real drunk, and does it again."

"Franklin, make sure it doesn't happen anymore. When you get back to San Pedro you should get Youth Protection in on it."

Adele stopped hitting the children, but she drank more heavily and became more sullen. After a few days, Franklin announced they were leaving: "We'll be heading back to San Pedro tomorrow. There's a cattle auction next week that I should be there for."

When he first arrived, Franklin had talked of staying a month or two. The visit had only been ten days. As Franklin was about to board his truck, he said: "Thanks for everything, Doc. Come down and see us soon."

"We will for sure," I answered.

It all sounded pretty hollow. I suddenly realized as they were pulling away that I should have taken Adele aside and talked to her, instead of leaving Franklin to deal with it inadequately. It was confusing. He was my guest, and she was his woman, and I felt it would be better if he handled it. But for the sake of those kids I should have tried. It might have been futile, but I should have tried. I'll make sure Franklin gets Youth Protection in on it. I'll call them myself if he doesn't. It's not easy being a doctor all the time. I wonder what it's like having a job you can stop at five o'clock and Saturday and Sunday. I sure blew that one.

The Noise in the Thicket

TOM WILLIS WAS A RETIRED FARMER in his seventies. He had worked for many years as the manager of a large commercial apple orchard before he bought his own farm. He still worked part-time planting and doctoring apple trees. When we bought our farm I hired him to help me plant some apple trees.

The planting took us a full day. Though the young trees were only two or three feet high, their roots demanded a hole several feet in diameter and several feet in depth. The roots had to be wrapped in burlap sacks to discourage mice from nibbling at them. After the trees were planted, Tom carefully explained the care they would require: constant watering in the first year, and yearly trimming. He explained how the trimming was critical. One had to acquire a feeling about branches; to sense which ones were going to bud, and which ones were going to drain energy and should be trimmed. He said for the first few years he would help us with the trimming.

Over the years Tom continued to care for the trees. He would come on his own to trim them without being called. Often he would just drop by to see how they were growing. He and his wife became patients in my practice.

Four years after I'd met him, Tom had a stroke which left his right arm and leg partially paralyzed. Three months after the stroke, he showed up to trim the apple trees. He walked with a cane. To get out across the fields to the trees he had to be supported on each side. He couldn't snip the branches himself anymore, but he could indicate with his cane where we should cut.

Over the next two years Tom developed Parkinson's disease. This gave him a tremor in both hands, an unsteady shuffling walk, a stooped posture, and a tightening of his face into a mask barely capable of reflecting emotions he was feeling.

A friend of mine who lived about forty miles away had an apple tree that was about twenty years old that had never blossomed well, and had never produced anything but a few maggoty apples. One day late in September, I told Tom about the problem my friend had with his tree, and he agreed to go and see it. I bundled him into my jeep, and drove the forty miles to my friend's place. Tom examined the tree and indicated with his cane which branches should be cut. As we worked, a cold autumn wind penetrated through our clothes. Dry leaves scraped along the ground.

That spring my friend's tree bloomed, and Tom withered. His lack of balance and difficulty in walking increased to the point where he spent most of his day lying on a couch in the living room. His wife, who herself now had severe arthritis, would prop him up and lead him to the kitchen and the toilet. She took exquisite care of him. He lay on the couch in clean pressed shirts and trousers. His hair was always combed, and he was clean shaven. But it was that spring that his mind began to go. His wife said that he might suddenly turn to her, as though they were still on their farm, and say something like: "I think we'd better sell that boar. He'll soon be too heavy to breed. The market's up right now. It would be a good time."

Much to her amazement, he seemed to reserve these kinds of lapses to times when they were alone, and seemed to be able to hold on to reality when friends were visiting. I only witnessed one of these lapses. It was autumn and I was making a last home visit before placing Tom in a chronic care hospital. His wife's arthritis had worsened and it was no longer possible for her to care for him.

That summer my friend's apple tree had produced a crop of wholesome apples. "Do you remember that friend of mine whose tree you trimmed last September?" I asked Tom.

"Sure," he answered. "Forty miles down there near Stanstead."

"He had a good crop of healthy apples this summer." I said.

"All it needed was trimming." Tom answered with a flicker of a smile forcing its way through his frozen Parkinsonian mask.

I was sitting in the living room writing a letter about Tom to the doctor in the chronic care hospital who would be taking care of him. Tom was lying on his couch in the living room. He was watching me write the letter. His gaze shifted for a minute to his rack of guns on the wall, then he turned to me and asked:

"Did you get a buck this year?"

Tom had always been an avid hunter.

"No, I don't really hunt anymore. I hunted in New Mexico when we lived among the Apaches, but I haven't since then."

Tom looked out the window and followed the course of some

leaves swirling across the lawn and said: "I got one. About a week ago. Right down on the road near your place. It was about seven in the morning. I was driving slowly along with a thirty-thirty on my gun rack, and I heard a noise in the thicket. I got that gun down as quick as a flash—and by the time he'd made his next move—I had him. He was a big one, with a seven point spread..."

"How are the Chickens?"

IT WAS ABOUT TEN-THIRTY at night. I was in my office talking to Diane Chreighton and her mother about Diane's anorexia. Diane was a fifteen-year-old girl who was always finding new ways to torment her family in retaliation for the ways in which she felt they were tormenting her. Refusing to eat was a new tactic in an old battle that I'd refereed many times.

Suddenly, as we were talking, we heard a loud squawking from our chicken house. I turned to Mrs. Chreighton and Diane and said: "You have a problem that is going to take quite a while to solve. That squawking you hear from the chicken house represents a problem I've had for five years that I could solve in five minutes. There's an animal who's been killing our chickens at night—"

"Go get him," said Mrs. Chreighton.

"We have lots of time," Diane added.

I knew they'd understand. They were farmers.

Every spring Lenore bought a hundred day-old chickens. Over the summer and fall she cared for them until they reached adult size. It was hard work. For the first few weeks they had to be fed and given water several times a day. The boys and I helped with feeding, and changing the straw in the chicken house, but Lenore was the driving force behind the operation. She taught herself about chicken feeds, just as she had in gardening, and just as she had in anything she turned her mind to. By late autumn, the chickens she raised were a colossal ten to twelve pounds in weight. They were more like turkeys than chickens. For five years now an animal had been sneaking into the chicken house and devouring several chickens per night. He would wait until August, when the chickens had reached an average of seven or eight pounds. Then he would strike every night.

Réjean's father Bertrand was an avid chicken raiser. He put it this way: "I've spent my life in chicken shit."

Lenore consulted with Bertrand about the problem of the chicken slayer. Despite Bertrand's eighty years in chicken shit he couldn't figure it out. He couldn't find a hole in the chicken house. He spent hours looking. Since he'd had that strange stroke which often caused him to burst into tears when he spoke, he would report to Lenore with a sob: "I can't find a hole. I don't understand it."

One night, in order to be there when the animal struck, Mark and Allen and several of their friends put up our tent beside the chicken house and slept in it. During the night they woke to the squawking, but in the time that it took for them to wake me, and for me to arrive with a gun—the animal was gone and had left two dead chickens. While Mark had come to wake me, the others saw "some kind of animal with large yellow eyes" slinking off in the darkness.

I left Diane and her mother and went down to the basement to get the deer rifle. I hadn't used it since we left San Pedro. A shotgun would have been more appropriate. A deer rifle was overkill, but it was all I had. I loaded six shells into the magazine. Lenore and the boys were watching television in the living room and hadn't heard the squawking. I told them what was happening so that they wouldn't be frightened by the shot. Mark and Allen wanted to come with me but I dissuaded them: "I'm not a good shot. If I miss we could have some kind of enraged animal on our hands. I'd rather he come after me and not you."

Rifle in hand, I ran down to the chicken house, pushed open the door, and switched on the light. An enormous raccoon holding a dead and bloody chicken glared at me with an expression of extreme annoyance. He was angry at being disturbed while eating.

I took aim and fired. A squawking hurricane of feathers, dust, straw, grain and chicken shit obscured my view as I looked for a dead raccoon. When the dust and feathers settled, I saw him sitting very much alive on a roof beam about two feet higher from where he had been initially. I aimed again and fired. I lost sight of him during another flurry of dust and feathers and then found him once again sitting very much alive on a higher roof beam. I fired a third short as he was starting to squeeze through a small hole behind the light fixture. It was covered by a hood over the light. That's how we had missed it all these years. This time I heard the bullet thud into his body. The expression on his face changed from anger to surprise and he fell to the floor. I felt sorry for him. It wasn't his fault. We had drawn him into our chicken house because of the hole in the roof. If there hadn't been a hole, he never would have bothered us, and I wouldn't have shot him.

Within a few months Diane was eating normally and went on to find other ways to torment her family. During the next year she got pregnant and gave the baby up for adoption. A few years later she drifted into Montreal and became heavily involved in drugs. She phoned me one day from Montreal and said she wanted help in getting off drugs. I arranged for her to enter a live-in drug rehabilitation programme. She failed the first time around but she's trying again. In a letter she sent me from the rehabilitation centre she wrote:

> ...As you said, my problems are going to take longer for me to solve than it took for you to deal with the problem in the chicken house, but I'm working on it. Many of the things we talked about that night, and things we've talked about other times, are helpful for me now in coming to understand more about why I do what I do. Most of all what helps is an assurance I always got from you that I was really worth something. That's something I didn't seem to get anywhere else.
>
> By the way, I gotta say it, I always felt sorry for that raccoon. It wasn't his fault that hole was there in the roof. It was yours. Sometimes I think about him lying there with that big wound in his belly from the deer rifle. It wasn't really fair. Anyway, how are the chickens? Hope they're O.K.
>
> Sincerely,
>
> Diane

The Big Bang

YESTERDAY STARTED like any other day. It didn't continue like one. The first patient was a woman I knew well whose husband had recently died of a stroke. She had suddenly lost her hearing on one side. Understandably she was terrified that she was having some kind of stroke. I was delighted to look inside her ear and find a huge blob of wax. I removed the wax and restored her hearing. She was delirious with relief.

That was a good case.

The second patient was a woman I knew well who always managed to come in with a new symptom shortly after I alleviated the last one. Today her problem was constipation. Her examination was normal. It always is. I spent a long time describing to her how she could modify her diet to get rid of constipation. As she was leaving she said: "Thank you very much doctor. I'll change my diet as you suggested. But I must tell you," she added, "when my bowels become regular I get weak."

You can't win. She was already telling me next week's symptom: weakness. I could hardly wait.

It all began with the third patient. I had never seen her before. She was from Montreal, and was visiting a relative who lived in the area. She was only going to be staying in the area for a few days.

"What's the problem?" I asked.

"I keep thinking there's going to be a big bang!" she answered. "It frightens me!"

"What do you mean? What kind of bang?" I asked.

"I don't know," she answered. "Just a big bang!"

She was completely overwhelmed with fear.

"Do you mean like the end of the world or—"

"I don't know. Just a big bang. I can't understand it."

I changed the subject and asked her about herself. She was the wife of a union official who did a lot of travelling. Since her children had left home she had found time heavy on her hands. The last child had moved out several weeks ago, and this had made her more aware of how alone whe felt. She wasn't suicidal. She wasn't hearing voices or having hallucinations. She wasn't waking early as some people do with depression.

"How do you and your husband get along?" I asked.

"We get along well," she said. "I guess I just find it hard to be alone so much now." She was returning to Montreal in the next few days.

"I think it has something to do with the loneliness," I said. "But why it's come down to this big bang I can't really say. I'm going to to give you the name of a psychiatrist in Montreal who can help you."

I gave her a few tranquilizers to take if she needed them until she saw the psychiatrist, and asked her to write me and let me know what happens.

I saw ten more patients. Then I saw Maurice Prevost. Maurice is a border guard who had bursitis in his shoulder. Pretty straightforward. I told him he should try physiotherapy along with anti-inflammatory medicine. He said he didn't have the time to go for physiotherapy. Two years ago another doctor had given him an injection of cortisone and it had gone away.

"But now it's back," I said. "That's what happens with cortisone. It often only helps temporarily. Physiotherapy takes more time and effort, but it's often curative."

"I understand, doc", Maurice said. "But there's no way I could get away from work these days. We're short-staffed. Give me the cortisone this time. Next time I'll go for physiotherapy."

"O.K., the patient's always right sometimes," I said. "But I have to warn you. Repeated injections of cortisone can sometimes weaken tissue. This is the second time you're getting a cortisone injection in that spot. Don't con anyone else into giving you any more."

I sat Maurice down on the examining table. Prior to injecting the cortisone, I injected some xylocaine to freeze the area. I inserted the needle and drew back to make sure I wasn't in a blood vessel. Xylocaine entering the circulatory system can cause cardiac arrest. I injected the xylocaine and reached for the cortisone. In that brief interval Maurice slipped to the floor, and his head struck it with a resounding bang.

It was the big bang the third patient had predicted, but it was happening to me—not to her.

Maurice was out cold. Lenore yelled up from the kitchen below: "What was that bang?"

"Nothing," I yelled back. "Somebody fell, but they're O.K."

"You sure? That was some bang!"

Maurice was far from O.K. He was still unconscious. I rolled him over onto his back to make sure he was breathing well and his heart was beating as it should. As I was taking his blood pressure, he began to stir. I was sweating. I had learned a lesson. I would never sit anyone up for an injection again. I would always make them lie down from now on.

"Where am I?" Maurice moaned.

"You're in my office. I was giving you an injection. You fainted and fell on the floor and hit your head."

"Who are you?" said Maurice.

"Your doctor," I answered limply. "Who are you?" I asked, dreading the answer I might get.

"Maurice Prevost," he answered. "But I don't know who you are or where I am. Wait. I know. I'm in Theroux's place. Yes, this is Theroux's place," Maurice said, as he got to his feet and looked out the window.

Now I really started to sweat. Theroux was someone who had owned my farm fifteen years ago. I was terrified. Poor Maurice! Poor me! I could see the headlines:

FALL FROM EXAMINING TABLE IN DOCTOR'S OFFICE; PATIENT SUFFERS PERMANENT AMNESIA.

I started to dial a neurologist at the University Hospital when Maurice turned to me and said:

"Doctor, what happened? You were about to give me an injection of cortisone—"

"That's it," I said gleefully. "Then you fainted and hit your head on the floor," I added with a big grin.

"How is your head? Let me see it."

"It hurts a bit in the back, but it's O.K."

There was a slight bump on the back of his head. His neurological exam was normal. There is a God.

"After your head hit the floor you were out cold for a few seconds. Then you had amnesia for a few minutes. You scared me to death."

"What about my cortisone injection?" Maurice asked.

"Are you kidding?" I answered. "You're going for physiotherapy," I said giving him a signed requisition. I'll give you a note for work also. They'll just have to let you go."

Later that day Lenore asked me:

"How did that patient slip?"

"Oh, it was an old lady. She just fell off her chair," I answered.

"Just like that? That's strange."

"Well no, she just sort of missed the chair."

I was exhausted. Later I would tell Lenore exactly what happened. But I just couldn't handle it now. I just wanted to forget about it. Until Maurice had finally come around and said my name, I had thought that Louis Watunda, the black magic medicine man from Fort Collins, had finally caught up with me for treating him for pneumonia against his will. While Maurice was pacing the floor and wondering where he was, I thought Louis Watunda had orchestrated the whole event, including the third patient's prediction of it. At the time, I vowed that if Maurice recovered his memory, I would get an honest job. Maybe I will someday.

"We thought you'd want to know"

THE PHONE RANG at about two in the morning. Again it was a long distance call from the States.

"This is the doctor speaking," I answered.

"Go ahead, caller," the operator said.

"Doctor, this is Mary Kanseah speaking." Mary was a nurse at San Pedro Hospital. I couldn't understand why she would be calling. "It's about Franklin——" she said hesitating.

"Yes? What's happened?"

"He had a brain hemorrhage. It came out of nowhere. He was dead within a half hour after it started. There was nothing they could do for him. We thought you'd want to know."

The next day we flew down to San Pedro for the funeral.

Franklin used to say: "When I die, I don't want a funeral. Just put me in a gunny sack and throw me over an arroyo." Pretty well everyone in San Pedro except the chief was at the funeral. The chief had always been jealous of Franklin's popularity. You may remember, that with Franklin in mind, and Franklin being of mixed Apache and Mexican origin, the chief had had a law passed that only full-blooded Apaches could be elected chief. A long procession of people placed gifts in Franklin's grave. A giant floral cowboy hat was placed on the grave to commemorate his creation of the tribal ranch.

As we were leaving the cemetery, I was thinking of Franklin's visit to Moe's river, and how despite the tension, our parting embrace had been real. The chief of police tapped me on the shoulder and said: "Don't ever think you're alone in the world." He came up beside me and added: "The Apache nation is behind you."

Code Five

Code Five

IT'S A HOT MORNING in July and I'm sitting in a small room with no
windows to the outside. There are four windows—but they are all
one-way glass that look into the examining rooms of the trainee doctors whom I'm supervising this morning. It's their first day. They are
just out of medical school and are beginning a two year training program as residents in family medicine. For a year now I've been working as a teacher in a university hospital. The hospital was built by the
Jewish community in Montreal at the turn of the century. It soon
became a teaching hospital for one of the city's oldest medical schools.
The hospital's Family Medicine Centre where I work and teach, began as a dispensary on the dock of the Montreal harbour, providing
medical care and social service for Jewish immigrants arriving from
Eastern Europe before and after World War One. In its present setting it is still essentially a dockside clinic because it services a densely
multi-ethnic district of the city called Côte-des-Neiges which could
be translated as "Hill of Snow," but never is. It is worth translating to
appreciate how the Southeast Asian, Indian, African, South American,
Caribbean and Middle Eastern immigrants feel when they look out
their windows on a snowy sub-zero day in February and wonder how
and why they got here. They arrived after the Second World War, and
along with the Greeks, Italians, and Portuguese who had already settled
in areas near the hospital, became our patients. They joined the English and French Canadians from across the city who chose our hospital for their medical care. Jews, particularly a large number of older
Jews who live in a maze of apartments near the hospital that form a
contemporary *shtetl*, are the final component in the mix of patients in
our clinic. I've loved the place from the first day; it's like going to
work every day in a Bazaar of World History. The cultural cross cur-
rents and intersections of time and place are staggering.

Half the time I teach and the other half I see patients. Right now
I'm watching as one of the residents introduces himself to his first
patient.

"My name is Dr. Swednicki," the resident says cheerfully. "What
brings you here this morning, Mr. Reynolds?"

Mr. Reynolds is about six feet two inches tall. His hair is in a pony tail. He is wearing a Hell's Angels' T-shirt, jeans, and motorcycle boots with chains. The bulging muscles of his arms and chest make his T-shirt look like a bandanna.

"I feel like I want to kill someone," Mr. Reynolds answers, looking straight across the desk at Dr. Swednicki.

Dr. Swednicki turns pale, begins to sweat and blurts out: "Who is it you're thinking of killing? Anyone in particular?"

"No one in particular," answered Mr. Reynolds, looking straight at Dr. Swednicki. "Just anyone."

"Excuse me," Dr. Swednicki says rising from his chair, "I'll be back in a minute."

Dr. Swednicki hastily fled his first patient and came around to see me in my room on the safe side of the glass. "What do we do now?" he asks.

"We call a CODE FIVE," I answer.

"What's that?" he asks.

"Watch," I answer.

I call the hospital switchboard and say: "CODE FIVE Room 407". I turn to Dr. Swednicki and explain: "In about two minutes five of the biggest and strongest orderlies in the hospital will be here. You and I will try and convince Mr. Reynolds to come and talk this over with the psychiatrist in the emergency room. If he refuses, four of these orderlies each grab a limb and the fifth grabs his head—and they carry him there. That's a CODE FIVE."

Mr. Reynolds went along willingly. I met him two days later when I was doing a shift in the emergency room. It's always bedlam down there. Patients are often kept in beds in the hallways surrounding the emergency room for days until a bed becomes free upstairs in the hospital. Except for the stretch between four a.m and eight a.m. there are almost always about thirty patients waiting to be seen in one of eight cubicles. In the middle of this chaos, while I was bent over a counter writing out some orders on a chart, someone tapped me on the shoulder. It was Mr. Reynolds: he was now wearing a blue bathrobe and slippers; he had two days growth of stubble on his face. I froze with fear. Those damn psychiatrists! They're so goddamn crazy — letting a killer walk around here for two days—was he going to take his revenge? It's moments like this that when I always wish I'd never treated Louis Watunda, that magic black medicine man, for pneumonia against his will.

"Got a match?" Mr. Reynolds asked.

While Dr. Swednicki had been seeing Mr. Reynolds, the three other residents were also seeing their first patients. One of the residents was seeing a gnarled old Jewish lady who had been a patient of the clinic for many years. Every two years she went through this change of doctors. The resident began wading through her enormous chart and asked:

"How old are you?"

He could have figured out her age himself by merely looking at her date of birth on the chart.

"Sonny, I am old," she answered.

The resident calculated her age from her date of birth. He wouldn't make that mistake again.

Another resident who was Italian was seeing an Italian patient. She was about twenty-four and attractive and he was in his early thirties and handsome. Since they were speaking Italian there was little point in my observing her. Whenever I did glance at her window, I noticed that they were talking animatedly and smiling and laughing. After an hour the resident came in to discuss the case: "He's depressed," she said.

The fourth resident was seeing a young Sri Lankan immigrant who had come for a first pre-natal visit. The patient was newly arrived in Canada and spoke no English. One of her relatives who spoke a little English was acting as her interpreter.

"How long have you been sexually active?" the resident asked, with one eye on a textbook opened at The Initial Exam in Pregnancy.

The interpreter repeated the question in Sri Lankan.

The young woman thought for a moment and answered.

The relative translated with a query in his voice: "Ten minutes?"

The resident who had seen the ageless old lady was now seeing a cocaine addict in his late twenties, who was telling him how he had managed to stop cocaine now for two weeks: "... After I had stolen from my older brother's fucken cash register, my little brother—he's only thirteen—said to me: 'Pietro what the fuck's the matter with you?' Then I knew I had hit the bottom. I had to stop. I had no choice. I wanted to get straight and make my fucken family proud of me..."

I had taken this teaching job in Montreal when Mark had reached high school age. If we had stayed in Moe's River, Mark would have had to travel by bus an hour and a half each way to get to a high school. Soon after Allen would have to do the same. Faced with that prospect we decided to move into the city. After so many years of wilderness and country living it was strange to be in a city: we missed the vast spaces we had been used to living in; we missed the people and the pace of country living; it was strange to go out your door and find yourself on a street with many houses. But it was hardest of all for Mark. He had gone through six years of Moe's River Elementary School with his friend Pete Winston and ten other kids being the only class in each succeeding grade. In Montreal he had entered a sprawling high school with hundreds of students and not known anyone. Most of the students were entering with at least a few friends whom they knew from elementary school. I remember leaving him at school the first day and the smile he tried to comfort me with as I drove off.

Mark had struggled like this when we moved from San Pedro to Moe's River. He knew that slowly new friends would happen. Then one of those nightmares that can suddenly materialize in the daytime at school occured. One day in the cafeteria at noon he accidentally bumped into one of the toughest kids in his grade. The tough kid's tray fell. He was furious. Because the accident had been Mark's fault he offered to pay for the food that had fallen. The tough kid took the money, and with his gang always at his side, he continued to extort money from Mark for weeks. So now not only did Mark have no real friends, but he had a gang after him. Mark, of course, forbade us from going to the principal.

"It would only make it worse," he said. "They're part of a gang that has kids in the upper grades. If I squeal they could get them on my case. Eventually they'll get bored with me."

We acquiesced to his reasoning but felt rotten and apprehensive about doing so. One afternoon Mark had a dentist appointment after school and Lenore picked him up at school to drive him there. As

Mark was getting into the car the tough kid and his gang spotted him. The tough kid picked up a large rock and threw it at the car. It hit the door on Mark's side and left a long scratch.

Lenore levitated from the car in a rage. She's quite small but muscular. She teaches aerobics and women's weight-lifting. She strode over to the tough kid and grabbed him by the collar of his windbreaker. She put her face up close to his and said: "Listen kid, you better get out of here before I kill you."

The tough kid was surprised. He was also scared. This lady wasn't big but she was crazy. His gang, including some of their girlfriends, and some bystanders who had seen him throw the rock, watched with intense interest to see what he would do. He turned away and walked off slowly.

"You better go faster than that," Lenore warned.

He went faster.

That night at home there was very little to say about what happened. Mark knew that Lenore had to do what she did. You can't let a kid throw a rock at your car. He also knew that now it was going to be worse for him. The next morning when I drove Mark to school, we didn't speak about what had happened and what might happen now. It was all we could think about but there was nothing to say. When we reached the school, Mark stepped out of the car and closed the door. I was just about to drive off, when he tapped the window. I rolled down the window to see what he wanted: "Dad," he said.

"Yes," I answered.

"I prefer to be cremated," Mark said, and smiled and turned and strode into the building.

Allen too was having his trials in turning from a country kid into a city kid and making new friends. It was a bit easier for a ten-year-old than a twelve-year-old but it was still nonetheless a constant struggle. Lenore and I had taken him to buy school clothes one Saturday morning when I noticed him eyeing a stylish overcoat. Generally he wore a hockey team jacket to school. He kept looking over the coat but couldn't seem to make up his mind about it. Suddenly he blurted out: "Could I get that coat? It's ninety dollars."

"If you're sure you like it and that you're going to wear it would be fine," I said. "What do you think, Lenore?"

"It's a warm coat. It's well made," Lenore said. "If you're sure your going to wear it, Allen, we'll get it.

We both couldn't imagine him wearing it.

A few days later I was driving Allen to hockey practice and he said: "Dad, you know that coat I bought? It's kind of cool, right?

"Right."

"Not the kind of thing I usually wear, right?"

"That's what I was thinking when we bought it. But I didn't say anything because I didn't want to interfere. You seemed to want it."

"Seemed to is a good way to put it," Allen said. "You know, this is a new place for me, this city. And I'm in a new school. Some of the older kids in school wear coats like that and I thought I'd try it."

"What happened when you wore it?"

"It worked."

"What worked?"

"Suddenly kids who never even let me know they thought I was alive were suddenly being friendly. There was one really pretty girl who's hardly ever said a word to me who asked me to let her borrow it at recess. I thought it was all pretty funny. I hadn't changed at all. I just put on a cool coat instead of my hockey jacket. But they all changed. It was really funny. I've gone back to my hockey jacket. I'm sorry for the ninety bucks."

"Don't worry about it." I said, "You thought you'd wear it. These kind of things happen to everybody. I think you learned a lot for ninety bucks."

Taking the teaching job had added another dimension to medicine for me. It seems that only a few years ago I was a frightened resident. Now I was teaching frightened residents. This morning one of the residents was a half-hour late and I had to see one of his patients. For that half-hour I was unavailable to the other residents as a supervisor.

"You're being late upsets the whole system," I explained to the resident. "It backs up three other doctors and their patients."

"I'm really sorry. But I couldn't find my stethoscope," the resident explained. "I kept thinking I'd find it any second and time kept going by."

"Next time come without it. People are counting on you," I said. "You could have borrowed one."

Later on in the day I misplaced my stethoscope and had to listen to a patient's chest. I wandered around the clinic looking for one I could borrow. I came across an examining room where the door was open. There was a patient sitting by the doctor's desk. The doctor must have stepped out and the patient was waiting for him to return. There was a stethoscope on the desk. The changeable name plaque on the door indicated that the resident who had been late this morning was using the room. He had probably gone to discuss the patient's case with a supervisor. I entered the room, excused myself to the patient, took the stethoscope and left a note on the table:

> This is what I do when I can't find my stethoscope. I'll bring it back in a few minutes.
>
> Thanks!

Recently another CODE FIVE occurred involving one of my patients. The patient was a young Jamaican immigrant who was brought here to work as a housemaid. She was homesick and being treated badly by her employers. She had also been jilted by her boyfriend shortly after undergoing an abortion. She had come in for insomnia and weight loss but it was clear that she was severely depressed and talked of suicide. With a lot of apprehension she agreed to see a psychiatrist in the emergency room. I explained her case to him and had to run off to one of my patients who had gone into labour. I returned to the emergency room after the delivery at around midnight to see what the psychiatrist had decided. I wondered whether she had been allowed to go home or had been hospitalized. I found her tied to a bed by her wrists and ankles. I was astounded at this development. The psychiatrist was gone. Another psychiatrist who was on call for the night was to see her in the morning. She explained to me what happened. The psychiatrist had assigned a medical student to do an initial interview. He had asked her a lot of questions such as: Do you know where you are? What's the date today? What year is it? What's a hundred minus seven? And seven from that? What does "People who live in glass houses shouldn't throw stones mean?" It's part of what's called a Mental Status Exam in the textbooks. Asked without a careful explanation of why you're doing it can certainly make someone feel you think they're crazy for sure. She had become discouraged by the interview and tried to leave. Because she had been classified as suicidal and forbidden to leave, a CODE FIVE was called. Five burly orderlies had jumped her and tied her to the bed.

I untied her.

"I'm really sorry about this," I said. "It's not what I had in mind when I said we'd get some help."

"I would hope so," she answered.

I called the psychiatrist on call for the night and explained what had happened. He was apologetic and came in immediately to see her. He was a doctor who had respect for people and listened to them. They got on well. He discharged her and made arrangements to follow her as a patient. As she was leaving she asked him: "Those doctors I saw this afternoon, are they psychiatrists?"

"Yes," the psychiatrist answered.

"I think you had better get some help for them," she said.

Sunset

Sunset

KUUDDJUARAPIK IS AN INUIT SETTLEMENT in Northern Quebec which is the end of the line for passenger jets. If you're travelling further north to the Arctic and sub-Arctic regions you travel on with Air Inuit on their smaller propeller planes. In winter (and it's winter ten months of the year up here) when you board an Air Inuit plane, it's so cold you can see your breath when you first get in. After a half hour of flying it starts to warm up, but when you're flying to Povungnituk, an Inuit settlement on the Hudson Bay coast that I often work at, the plane stops every three-quarters of an hour or so at other settlements along the route, and you lose what heat you've gained as they open the cargo doors and let in the cold air once again. Kuuddjuarapik has a few other names which people use according to their perspective: it is also known as Great Whale among the English; Poste-de-la-Baleine among the French; and as Whapamagustui among the Cree.

Right now I'm sitting in the coffee shop in the airport at Kuuddjuarapik. That's kind of a joke because the airport is a one-room shack, and the coffee shop is another tiny shack about twenty yards from the airport—which at thirty-below zero is a considerable distance. The coffee shop is owned by two old Inuit ladies who have great smiles but make lousy sandwiches with stale bread. You wash the stale sandwiches down with weak coffee laced with canned milk. The shop has a name in Inuktitut, the language of the Inuit, written on the door. It says *Tukvik*. I have stopped here many times over several years, but it had never occurred to me to ask what the word means. It had never occurred to me to ask, because having worked among the Inuit for several years, I knew how they always seem uncomfortable with direct questions about anything. Everybody is expected to learn by observation rather than by asking. When you ask a direct question, you usually get an evasive answer. But suddenly I wanted to know what this word meant on the door of the coffee shop. As one of the ladies handed me a stale sandwich I boldly asked: "What does *Tukvik* mean?"

The Inuit lady never stopped smiling, but she looked as if she'd been shot. This was an enormous imposition. The Inuit call white people *Quallunaat*. It literally means "bushy eyebrows" but you can't pin any Inuit down on the real meaning. We'll never really know what it means. This Inuit lady never stopped smiling, but she was probably thinking: *Damn this Quallunaat! Why doesn't he just eat his stale sandwich like all the others, and not bother me with this kind of question?* It took her several minutes to think about the question before she answered it. She was really struggling with it. A bead of sweat trickled down her forehead. She took out some tobacco and cigarette paper, and rolled herself a cigarette. She took a few puffs, and just as I'd about given up hope and figured she wouldn't answer, she smiled and said: "Maybe it means a place where you only stop a moment."

Maybe is an important word among the Inuit. It's used in a way that makes sure you allow everyone the maximum freedom to make their own decisions. For example: "Doctor, someone says they saw a wolf today on the road to your house. When you go home from the hospital tonight, maybe you should take the back road."

It's up to you. I'm just telling you something that it's useful for you to know. Do what you want. That is the spirit in which the old lady prefaced her definition of *Tukvik*, the name on the coffee shop with "maybe it means". "Maybe", because maybe someone else could describe it better; and because maybe it's a question and answer that's bigger than both of us — and nobody can really answer it adequately.

The airport is a one-room shack. There's one bench on the wall opposite the ticket counter. The bench only seats a small fraction of the people milling around the room. There are always lots of people milling around the room because they're waiting for planes that are late or grounded because of snowstorms or fog. The waiting people trundle back and forth between the coffee shop and the airport. The Inuit are prodigious smokers. Both shacks are filled with smoke. They are also prodigious gum chewers. So someone is either blowing smoke in your face or cracking gum in your ear. There are dogs in crates barking at one another. There are policemen escorting handcuffed prisoners south to do jail terms. There are patients on stretchers being transported to southern hospitals. The two shacks have one virtue. They are warm from being overcrowded. In the north warmth is the name of the game. When you come out of a cold plane either of those two shacks is heaven. You don't care who's blowing smoke or cracking gum.

In the toilet, along with the usual obscenities seen anywhere (although this is the only place where I've seen SHIT spelled SIHT) are some heartfelt messages like this one from a woman with a Cree name to a man with an Inuit name that reflect the fact that Kuuddjurarapik is a place of passage:

Qualingo Putugu
Come back to Great Whale River
I miss you
                    Irene Otter Eyes

On a shelf behind the ticket counter there is a pile of Air Inuit sweatshirts for sale. For several years now I've been trying to buy some for Lenore and the boys. Each time I approach the ticket agent and ask about buying some, I've gotten an answer something like this:

"Look, Mac, I haven't got time for that stuff! If the fog lifts I'm going to have two 737s coming in almost at the same time. Then there's the ambulance plane that the Twin Otter has to meet at LG-2. I don't know how they expect me to sell that stuff while I have to run an airport where everything has to be rescheduled at least five times."

As you can gather, I like the airport at Kuuddjuarapik. Being stranded here in a storm or fog is one of those moments where I can drop out. I can't be reached; I'm not responsible for anything. Today I'm heading back down to Montreal. It's been seven years now since we moved from Moe's River to Montreal. I first started travelling to Povungnituk several years ago when the director of the hospital there phoned the medical school and told them they were desperately short of doctors. The medical school, knowing I had previously worked in native health, asked me if I were willing to help. I began going up for several weeks four times a year, and in addition to working there myself, had it designated as a rural teaching site for our residents to work in. It turned out well for Povungnituk and for the medical school. It's a good training experience for the residents, and they do provide some help for the manpower shortage, as one of them is now always on rotation there. Quite a few of the residents have taken jobs there when they graduate.

Of course, the plane is late. I've been lucky enough to get a seat at a table in the coffee shop, which enables me to write a letter to Martin in Kenya. I am writing him about the plight of the Inuit teenagers who often feel hopelessly caught between two cultures and find the problems of unemployment and family breakdown more than they can deal with: "…Sometimes it feels like you're working in a war zone: The hospital van (it's not really an ambulance) pulls in with a teenager who has shot himself and is bleeding to death. Often they've been sniffing gas or are drunk but sometimes they're not. Many times it's a shotgun wound in the belly. The kid is clutching at the wound and moaning —"

People are starting to move from the coffee shop over to the airport. Maybe (as the Inuit say) the plane is coming. I better find out. I put my unfinished letter to Martin in my briefcase and make the twenty yard dash in thirty-below cold over to the airport. A snowstorm is building up. In the airport people are milling around, smoking and cracking gum. There is a vague rumour circulating that a plane will be arriving in twenty minutes, but it isn't official. The ticket agent is too beside himself to ask him. He would probably answer: "Look Mac, I'm not sure. And even if it comes, there's probably not enough visibility for it to land."

Writing Martin about the teenagers in Povungnituk makes me think of my own teenagers. Mark is now nineteen and Allen is seventeen. I think of a wedding in Moe's River we were invited to a few weeks ago. One of the Winston boys was marrying a girl from another family who were also former patients of mine. We hadn't been to Moe's River for five years. We stayed with Lorraine, my former secretary. While we sat around talking to Lorraine and her family, Mark drove over on his own to see his friend Pete Winston. They were both nineteen now. They hadn't seen each other since they were fourteen. Mark described it to me this way: "As I drove up, he and his dad and some of his brothers were just coming out of the barn. They were just finishing the morning milking. At first I could tell they didn't recognize me. They probably thought I was some kind of city slicker who was going to try and sell them something. They looked kind of disdainful. Then all of a sudden Pete smiled and said: 'You must be kidding—'"

They embraced and Mark came back with barn smell on him.

The day after the wedding we visited Réjean. As always, he showed the boys his latest newborn calves and piglets—just as he had done throughout their childhood. While we were in his barn, I noticed Franklin's fender-jack leaning against a wall, and I remembered Franklin giving it me on the day we left San Pedro. I had given it to Réjean when we had moved to the city.

Mark. Nineteen! I visited him a few weeks ago in the physiology lab at the university. He is studying physiology and has a part-time job as a medical research assistant. It is at the end of the afternoon. He shows me the experiment he is working on. Through the window of the lab the lights of the city below us and the lights of the bridges over the river glow luminously—just as they did in my student days. The difference here is that Mark as a student is doing scientific research that I can only marvel at and couldn't do. I watch him pouring, decanting and titrating solutions into machines, and might as well be witnessing a religious ceremony: my comprehension is minimal; my reverence is total.

Mark is working with some other physiology students who like himself are applying to medicine and hoping to get in. At a moment when they are taking a break at the window he introduces me to them: "This is my dad," he says. "He's a doctor..."

Allen at seventeen. The eight year old who used to muse about "space having no end and just going on forever" is now on his way to becoming a physicist and ponders over these types of questions in mathematical terms drawn from quantum mechanics. He valiantly tries to explain these concepts to me in layman's terms, but all I can do is marvel happily at his comfort with the complexity I can't even begin to fathom.

I remember watching Franklin sitting in his pick-up truck with his two grown sons that morning in San Pedro when they drove off to kill the rattlesnake, and wondering what it would be like when my sons were grown older. I'm even prouder and happier that I'd imagined I would be.

An hour later a plane approached the airport, but the storm increased in the interval, and visibility was too poor for it to land. Four hours later, after the storm subsided, the plane returned and we were able to board and take off. Now we're about twenty minutes out of Montreal and I'm thinking about an old Inuit who is sitting with his daughter across the aisle from me. His name is Moses Novalinga. I had seen him as a patient several days earlier in Povungnituk. He has cancer of the bowel, and I arranged for him to be treated in Montreal. It looked as if his tumour was well localized and not spread. If that turns out to be true, he might never have a recurrence of the cancer after surgery. He was eighty-one years old. The average length of life among the Inuit is fifty-six years compared to seventy-six years in the south. The difference is not due so much to disease, as to violence, accidents, and alcohol. The Inuit who reach eighty-one are usually the ones who have a strong adherence to the old ways. They are the ones who have kept up the tradition of fishing and hunting, and struggled to keep their families intact. This man was one of these patriarchal figures. He had lived the most active part of his life as a hunter in the days when the Inuit still lived as nomads. He had roamed the ice floes and lived in igloos in the time before permanent settlements were established. I had watched him as we took off from Povungnituk early that morning. I saw him straining at his window to keep the tiny settlement in view as it disappeared into an endless expanse of snow-covered ground.

"How's your dad doing?" I asked his daughter, who was going along as his escort.

"Fine." She answered. "He's never been in a plane before."

I could only guess at some of the emotions Moses felt as we pulled away from Povungnituk. I have been in many planes, but I'm always stunned by that particular take-off. As the two pilots place their hands on the throttle, the engine roars, and the plane lifts above the settlement, you're instantly confronted with either an endless expanse of snow in winter, or an endless expanse of sea, rock and tundra in summer. Suddenly you become aware again of the immensity surrounding the life you were living down there in that little village, and the infinite immensity of the universe surrounding life on this planet— and for that moment you remember you're part of that infinity.

We're now pulling into the outskirts of Montreal. It's five o'clock and the sun is going down. I'm watching Moses as he looks out his window. Now you can make out miles of buildings, streetlights and bridges—all flashing under a haze of smoke. I had watched him all the way down from Povungnituk, as we passed successively through the barren grounds, the forest areas and the farming regions. He had observed it all with intense interest and equanimity. But now as we flew over this haze of smoke, lights and endless rows of buildings, I saw him begin to look alarmed. He was sitting erect, and glancing from one window to another, in what seemed to be disbelief that they all could be revealing an endless expanse of the same objects: lights, streets, buildings, and bridges—all under the same smokey haze. At this point, the old man turned to his daughter and asked her something in Inuktitut. He had hardly spoken during the whole journey. I was curious to know what he had said. At that moment the daughter turned to me and smiled.

"My father just asked me, are all these houses?"

It's 2:00 a.m. and the phone is ringing in one of those houses Moses Novalinga saw from the plane. The house is mine and the voice on the phone is a resident from the hospital:

"Doctor, we've just admitted a patient of yours named Selma Evans, who went into labour about 10:00 p.m. She's five centimetres dilated and her contractions are strong—"

"Sorry," I interjected, "I'm in Povungnituk. You'll have to call whoever—"

"Dad," interrupted Allen, who was studying late and had picked up another phone in the house at the same time as I did, "you're dreaming—"

I woke up abruptly. "Sorry," I said to the resident, "I just flew in from Hudson Bay a few hours ago. I started out from there at five in the morning. It's been a long day. I'll be there in twenty minutes.

I dressed hurriedly in the dark, not wanting to wake Lenore. Often when I dress this way, later in the day I find myself wearing two different coloured socks. As I dressed I wished I was in Kuukjuarapik stranded in the airport by a snowstorm. But once I was really awake and driving to the hospital with a song called "Country Road" playing on an all night radio show I was glad to be where I was—on the way to deliver the first child of a couple in their early twenties, who I had known since they were in highschool. As I drove through the deserted streets to the hospital with memories of other early morning car and ambulance rides in San Pedro and Moe's River, and early morning medivac flights up north, I was glad Selma had waited until I was back to go into labour.

5:15 a.m.

I'm back home and writing a very short note in my journal before I crawl back into bed and go where the pinballs go between games, and pray that no one else lights up the board because I've got to get up by seven to be at work by eight. The delivery went well. A small creature recently fish and now resembling Selma and Larry, emerged blood-stained and glistening, and began to breath and cry and move its limbs— a sight the doctor is grateful to behold. I'm always stunned at the tiny hand—the fingers unfolding with real fingernails.

I left Larry happily sitting at the bedside holding a baby girl of six pounds in his large arms, and Selma sleeping with a smile on her face.